The Health Care Supervisor's Guide to Cost Control and Productivity Improvement

Charles R. McConnell

The Genesee Hospital
Rochester, New York

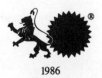

AN ASPEN PUBLICATION®
Aspen Systems Corporation

1986

Rockville, Maryland
Royal Tunbridge Wells

Library of Congress Cataloging in Publication Data

McConnell, Charles R.
The health care supervisor's guide to cost control and productivity improvement.

"An Aspen publication."
Includes bibliographies and index.
1. Health facilities—Business management. 2. Medical care—Cost effectiveness.
3. Health services administration. I. Title. [DNLM: 1. Cost Control—methods.
2. Efficiency. 3. Health Facility Administrators. WX 157 M4785h]
RA971.3.M355   1986   362.1'1'0681   85-26831
ISBN: 0-87189-254-5

Editorial Services: Jane Coyle

Library of Congress Catalog Card Number: 85-26831
ISBN: 0-87189-254-5

Printed in the United States of America

1 2 3 4 5

*For Kate, and for Rick, Mike, Kelly,
Matt, and John. Thanks, special people.*

Table of Contents

Preface

Few if any supervisors have escaped hearing the common observation that "A hospital (or almost any other health care organization) should be run like a business." Surely most persons voicing this contention mean to suggest that organizations in the business of providing health care need to become more businesslike in their affairs, especially as concerns finances. But other, more subtle beliefs are conveyed when someone says, "A hospital should be run like a business."

Consider the word *like*. The most straightforward meaning of this word is *resembling closely* or *similar to*; resembling but not identical, similar but not the same. Thus implicit in "A hospital should be run like a business" is a differentiation between them—a hospital is a hospital and a business is a business, but it would be beneficial if the former were run more like the latter.

Certainly many people in health care have trouble equating hospital and business. Just as surely they have difficulty thinking of the health care industry as a legitimate entity because they separate the concept of health care from that of industry. Health care is healing and altruism but industry is smokestacks and profits. One is giving and the other is taking. Perhaps closer to the truth would be, "A hospital should be run *as* a business." Essentially meaning *in the same manner or way*, the word *as* provides a stronger sense of sameness linking hospital and business. However, an implication of separateness remains.

The last vestiges of differentiation vanish only when one can concede, in all honesty, that a hospital *is* a business. A hospital or any other health care organization is indeed a business. It may differ markedly from the business of, for example, selling automobiles, manufacturing radios, growing grain, or providing consulting services. However, as long as it generates income by providing something that people desire, it is a business.

The point of the foregoing word play is, of course, to suggest that a health care organization is a business and ought to be run in the way a business should be run if it is to succeed at what it was formed to accomplish. Nevertheless, *business* remains a negative term to many in health care—workers and supervisors alike.

Another negative term, if not actually a dirty word, to many in health care is *profit*. Even those who accept the necessity for a not-for-profit entity to finish each year with an excess of income over expenses—for example, most finance directors, chief executive officers, and trustees—tend to refer to profit as *operating surplus* or some similarly euphemistic label. Yet there is nothing in not-for-profit corporation law to suggest that such an organization may not make a profit (the laws dictate only that the surplus generated by a not-for-profit corporation cannot accrue to the benefit of any private individual or group).

Indeed, it is becoming widely recognized that a not-for-profit health care organization *must* make a profit to maintain long-run viability. How else is an insitutition continually to replace its buildings and equipment in the presence of normal inflation?

The business of maintaining and improving health and preserving life places health care organizations in a unique category among businesses. However, this category—the health care industry—is now subject to many of the same forces and pressures that have long had an impact on other industries. Specifically:

- different pricing structures and varying payment methods have created price competition among providers of health care;
- competition has been further intensified by an oversupply of health care resources (such as excess beds) in some areas;
- alternatives to hospitalization and to other forms of care are developing rapidly and provide still another competitive dimension;
- those who ultimately pay for most health care—employers, individuals (as taxpayers as well as patients), and government—are rebelling against ever-increasing costs.

As a result, health care organizations are being forced to adopt as a real goal to be pursued very seriously that which they have long espoused only as a stated goal: To deliver quality care in a cost-effective manner.

The literature of health care management has recently exploded with advice on how to meet the new financial and competitive challenges. However, most of this advice is aimed at the upper levels of health care management. Certainly the task of top management is difficult; this group must point out the direction and set the pace, and for the most part they are operating in dim light at best. Critical decisions must be made and important new policies established, but it is those managers below the top echelon in the hierarchy—the greatest number of managers in any organization—who must implement these decisions and policies.

The Health Care Supervisor's Guide to Cost Control and Productivity Improvement is designed specifically for the first-line supervisor and middle manager. It is for the manager of an organizational subunit, the manager who must make the day-to-day operating decisions that translate top management's direction into effective action.

This volume recognizes the reality of the supervisor's position. For the most part first-line supervisors are not accountants or finance experts (where cost control is concerned) and are ordinarily not industrial engineers (where productivity improvement is concerned). The book also recognizes that the supervisor's authority is limited to the boundaries of his or her own department. With these limitations in mind, and while providing fundamentals of certain topics for overall understanding, this book focuses on:

- those actions that the individual supervisor can take to control costs and improve productivity;
- those conditions or practices for which the supervisor can suggest and inspire positive change in other elements of the organization;
- those positive attitudes which, when adopted by the supervisor and evidenced in supervisory behavior, can spread to the work group and to other organizational elements.

In short, *The Health Care Supervisor's Guide to Cost Control and Productivity Improvement* helps the supervisor determine what to do, where to go for assistance, and how to inspire cost consciousness in the work group. It has long been recognized in business that the most effective policies are those that are reasonable, rational, and strongly supported from the top down. Equally deserving of recognition is the reality of practice—that the most effective implementation often occurs from the bottom up. With regard to cost control and productivity improvement, the size of the buck may be determined on high, but the buck stops where the action resides—on the desk of the first-line supervisor.

Part I

Cost Containment: Now and Ever After

Chapter 1

Cost Control as a Way of Life

To welcome a problem without resentment is to cut it in half.

Anonymous

Might just as well forget your old troubles; there are more coming.

Anonymous

Chapter Objectives

- Examine the possible causes of the rapid increase in health care costs.
- Identify the primary sources of cost containment pressure applied to health care institutions.
- Consider likely future directions of health care providers in the face of permanent change in the fiscal environment.
- Establish the role of the individual supervisor in cost control and productivity enhancement.

THE BALLOONING HEALTH CARE BILL

It is no secret to people who work in health care or to those who deal with the health care industry only as consumers that health care costs are increasing. Neither is it unknown to most persons that health care costs are rising at a faster rate than most other costs of living and are consuming an ever-expanding share of the nation's total resources. The nation's population is enjoying generally better health and longer life than ever before and receiving better health care than has ever been available to the citizens of any country, but it is paying for these unquestioned benefits at a dramatically increasing rate.

In 1960, total health care expenditures in the United States amounted to approximately 5.5 percent of the gross national product (GNP). By 1980, health care expenditures as a percentage of GNP had grown to approximately 9.5 percent. During the same 20 years, 1960 to 1980, total United States health care expenditures rose from about $30 billion to approximately $250 billion per year. In 20 years the national health care bill had multiplied more than eight times. During the same 20-year period hospital room rates increased by more than 600 percent and physicians' fees rose by more than 300 percent.[1]

The total population of the United States increased markedly from 1960 to 1980. However, per capita health care expenditures have increased at a rate far outstripping the increase in the number of people. In 1960, per capita health care expenditures in the United States were $146.30. By 1980, annual health care expenditures had risen to an average of $1,067.06 for every man, woman, and child in the United States.[2]

A disturbingly high level of health care cost is not simply a spectre that might appear but is already present in a number of dimensions. In late 1983, former secretary of Health, Education, and Welfare, Joseph Califano, stated that:

- Health care costs account for more than ten percent of the gross national product.
- Health care expenses exceed defense outlays as the fastest-growing portion of the federal budget.
- Health care costs—not income taxes—are the biggest item in the difference between an employer's total compensation costs for an employee and the amount of pay that employee takes home.[3]

Health care costs in the United States are increasing at a rate roughly double the national rate of inflation. It is estimated that by 1990 the national health care bill will have reached $8.5 billion per year—on the average, $3,700 per year for every person living in the United States.[4] A frequently asked question is: What are the causes of this seemingly runaway escalation of health care costs? Do they lie primarily in medical advances of such compounding sophistication that more complex skills, more exotic drugs, and more expensive equipment are constantly required to gain ground in the endless struggle to preserve health and prolong life? Do at least some of the causes lie in the waste and inefficiency of a highly fractionated health care delivery system? Or are health care costs so high because people who do not have to pay their own health care bills out of pocket are overusing health care services, or because some providers are reaping unconscionable profits? Is it a combination of these and more causes that drives up the cost of health care at an alarming rate?

Most people have opinions about the reasons for the rapid rise in health care costs, and some argue their opinions convincingly and at great length. However, it is evident that arguments alone and even arguments plus limited action have done little to stem the alarming rate of increase in health care costs.

Forces Fueling Health Care Cost Inflation

The generally acknowledged causes of health care cost inflation, both real and perceived, include:

- increased hospital day rates, stemming from increases in the cost of providing all hospital services and supporting the delivery of those services;
- increased use of laboratory tests, x-rays, drugs and pharmaceuticals, and other ancillary services, and their increased cost;
- increases in the number of procedures prescribed medically for each patient, including significant increases in the total number of operations performed;
- steady increases in physicians' charges;
- overexpansion of hospital facilities and duplication of hospital facilities and services;
- advancing medical technology as increasingly more sophisticated equipment and skilled labor are used in health problems and more resources are applied to specific emerging medical needs of the population;
- increasingly larger and more numerous malpractice settlements, and corresponding increases in malpractice insurance premiums for provider organizations and individual medical practitioners alike;
- increasing costs of operating various government agencies as those agencies become more involved in regulating health care quality and cost;
- alleged overuse of the health care systems by some consumers, and the supposed abuse of some medical insurance programs.

It is popular practice for the various participants in the health care system—individual providers, provider organizations, payers, regulators, and consumers—to blame each other for the largest part of the increase; the reality of the total increase remains to be reckoned with. Ultimately, however, it is the health care provider, whether individual or institution, who is required to deal most intimately with growing health care costs.

Cost Containment Pressures

A number of pressures, some independent of each other but most inter-related, bear on the institutional provider of health care. Health care institutions are receiving clear indications of means to slow the rate of growth in the health bill and to contain costs. These pressures are being applied by:

- employers, who pay a large share of increasing health care costs through their payment of health insurance premiums and the direct costs of company-sponsored health plans;
- government, which pays a significant share of increasing health care costs with tax revenues;
- labor unions, many of which see their members losing ground in the area of health benefits by having to bear directly a larger portion of increasing health care costs;
- consumer groups, collectives of citizens reacting to dramatic increases in the cost of an essential service;
- taxpayer groups, collectives of citizens who see their taxes related to health care increasing without equivalent increases in benefits received.

All of the foregoing pressures bear on the health care provider, the individual health care institution. The individual institution remains charged with the task of providing top-quality health care, including the provision of all new technology that could possibly have a positive impact on the restoration of health and the protection and extension of life while containing the increase in health care costs.

Although cost containment pressures are directed at the institution as a whole, within the health care institution these pressures must ultimately come to bear on those individuals who actively control or influence the expenditure of health care dollars. Specifically, cost containment pressures are ultimately focused on the point at which ground-level action must be taken to control costs, the individual department manager or cost center supervisor.

EMPLOYER REACTION TO SPIRALING COSTS

From the mid-1960s or earlier until the early 1980s, many employers left the management of health care costs primarily to health insurance carriers. The majority of health insurance premiums were established by a standard markup over the long-run cost of claims, so insurance carriers profited from increasing health care costs (since a percentage markup applied to a larger base yields a larger profit). In terms of how insurance carriers operated, there appeared to be an incentive to provide more and costlier service and thus a lack of incentive to adopt cost-saving practices.

Employers pay the largest share of the health care bill through health insurance premiums on behalf of employees. Health insurance costs were once a budget item of no particular importance to most business organizations, but because of dramatic increases in health care costs, this is no longer the case. Health insurance premium costs are now major items of cost to most companies.

During 1982 and 1983, inflation of health care costs occurred at the rate of 15 to 20 percent.[5] With this double-digit inflation, corporate and public employers began to feel the financial pinch associated with health care costs and began to shift more of these costs to their employees. As a result, during 1982 and 1983, increases in health insurance premium costs borne by employees averaged 20 to 40 percent.[6]

Overall, efforts of employers to reduce the budgetary impact of escalating health care insurance premium costs have included:

- increasing the share of the premium costs for employees who pay a portion of their own health insurance coverage through payroll deduction;
- establishing an employee share of the health insurance premium cost where none existed before;
- calling for employees to bear the full impact of future increases in health insurance premiums, thus requiring employees to pay an increasing proportion of premium costs as these costs grow;
- establishing absolute dollar caps on employer contributions;
- requiring employees to pay larger health plan deductibles.

All of the foregoing serve to pass an ever larger part of the increasing financial burden of health care on to employees, with employees generally being required to pay more and more of their care coverage.

Actions that may be seen by many companies as part of their necessary cost containment efforts are viewed by employees as direct losses of disposable income. Further, in unionized companies such actions are seen by bargaining units as the intended result of take-away bargaining, which has the effect of shifting the burden of health care premium costs from employer to employees.

Thus, the direct impact of employer reactions to spiraling health care costs has meant heightened awareness of the health care cost issue. The intense interest of all concerned parties is rising because of a most effective stimulus to education on the part of both employers and employees—direct impact on the pocketbook.

EMPLOYEE RESPONSE TO HEALTH BENEFIT COST CUTTING

It is certainly not unusual for someone who once received something free of charge but who must now pay for it, or who sees the accustomed cost of basic coverage or service increasing markedly, to react with complaints. The recent history of rapid health care cost increases and numerous employers' responses to such increases have caused many individual voices to be added to the general outcry concerning health care costs. In many instances, cost increases and employer responses have given rise to the vocal objections of labor unions.

To a considerable extent, labor unions are in the forefront of organized opposition to the shifting of health insurance premium increases to employees. In December 1983, the Service Employees International Union (SEIU) announced the commencement of a national effort to counter rising health care costs and oppose what has been described as increasing management attacks on health care benefits. This union has gone on record as pressing to link Blue Cross and Blue Shield premium rates to formal cost containment efforts and has also proposed to freeze physicians' fees.[7]

The SEIU has identified ten states as targets for its efforts: California, Georgia, Illinois, Michigan, Missouri, New York, Ohio, Oregon, Pennsylvania, and Texas. The union will encourage passage of legislation aimed at freezing rates and fees until insurers can meet specific cost containment standards and until reasonable physicans' fee schedules can be negotiated with doctors. The union elected to focus efforts at the state legislative level because of the belief that the federal government has consistently refused to adopt cost containment legislation nationally.

Other unions have been invited to join SEIU in the effort to work toward retaining workers' health care coverage through tougher collective bargaining and through more direct involvement in working for the passage of regulatory legislation. In general, the unions have pointed out that:

- There are no solid plans in the works to cap physicians' fees.
- There is essentially no limit on capital expansion and on equipment purchases by providers, except in a very few states.
- There are inadequate requirements for insurance carriers to adopt cost-saving practices.

Much of the union position suggests that true health care cost containment will require:

- more efficient administration of insurance plans than currently prevalent;
- discontinuance of unnecessary medical procedures;
- vastly increased use of alternatives to hospitalization;
- adoption of flat fee schedules and competitive bidding for "hospitals, clinics, medical groups, and individual doctors."[8]

Overall, most unions can be expected to engage in considerably tougher bargaining in regard to health care benefits with the general objective not to acquire further gains but rather to prevent further losses.

Unions and other employee and consumer groups, plus selected arms of government and certain interested health care providers, are encouraging the health care system to turn toward:

- increasing emphasis on preventive medicine;
- use of mandatory second opinions regarding the necessity of surgery;
- further shifting to the use of alternatives to hospitalization;
- means of further reducing the length of hospital stays;
- organized enhancement and support of self-help programs to assist people in dealing with hypertension, alcoholism, diabetes, and other chronic ailments;
- implementation of new programs intended to reduce and control occupational health and safety hazards.

Relative to a working individual's earnings, health care coverage costs for many employees are no longer negligible. As these costs are a major and growing budget item for businesses, so are they a cost element of increasing concern for individuals, who are deeply concerned over health care costs and will continue to be concerned, especially as long as these costs grow out of proportion to growth in other costs of living.

THE FOCUS OF COST CONTAINMENT PRESSURE

Some people feel that any organization or individual that renders bills for providing any service related to health is automatically responsible for at least part of the general cost escalation problem. Most frequently tagged with such responsibility are the direct, hands-on providers of health care services, both organizations and individuals, and especially hospitals and physicians.

The hospital is frequently seen as a complex organization that continually and wholly arbitrarily charges more for a vital service that is required by people who have few if any alternatives to using that service. The hospital is often seen as a rich organization; critics do not understand how this organization could absorb such large sums of money without having plenty left over. It is not unusual for a hospital's credibility regarding its true financial state to be low in the view of many users of its service.

Physicians are seen by many as high-income earners who arbitrarily charge more for the provision of a vital service that is required by people who have few alternatives. In brief, the hospital and the physician are both frequently seen as charging more solely because their services are essential and there are no ready alternatives.

Certainly hospital and physician costs are necessarily the cost elements of greatest concern in the health care system. In 1980, hospital charges accounted for 40.3 percent of all health care expenditures in the country, by far the largest share of the health care dollar. During the same year, physician charges accounted for 18.9 percent. By comparison, the third largest component of cost in 1980 was nursing home care, which consumed 8.4 percent of the health care dollar.[9]

It was once unthinkable that serious steps would ever be taken to cap health care expenditures, actually to place a limit on the amount of money flowing into the system. Capping, it was reasoned by many, would inevitably lead to cutbacks in service and to the erosion of the quality of health care. However, capping health care expenditures is now being done by various reimbursement regulations. Indeed, reimbursement regulations imposed on the system have one major ultimate net effect: They force changes to occur within by limiting the inflow of the system's primary resource, the money required to operate.

In a number of ways external regulation has guaranteed chaos within the system. Consider thousands of hospitals and tens of thousands of other providers, all participating in a loosely defined "system" composed of countless cottage-industry elements and supported entirely by seemingly runaway cost inflation. Pressure is then applied by capping the cost of the system and limiting the rate of cost growth by regulating the input of the system's critical resource. The numerous elements making up the system respond to this pressure in a variety of ways:

- Some providers change the character of services they provide or particular markets they serve. For example, a particular hospital feeling the financial pinch might abandon the maternity service, a money-losing service perhaps more efficiently provided by another institution, and concentrate on same-day surgery.
- Some providers, unable to adjust to the changing financial environment, may voluntarily or involuntarily go bankrupt and eventually leave the system.
- Some providers may merge or otherwise affiliate with other providers, reducing the total number of health care provider organizations but adding to the total number of institutions involved in a multi-hospital system.
- Some providers may take steps to achieve higher levels of internal operating efficiency so as to adjust to the decline in the rate of growth of financial resources available.

Drastic changes have occurred in the United States health care system since external pressure began to be applied to hospitals. In 1968, there were 7,991 hospitals in the country. By 1979, the number had dropped to 7,085, a decline of 11.3 percent in 11 years.[10] Further change is expected in the number of active hospitals. It has been estimated, for example, that the impact of the federal government's diagnostic related group (DRG) reimbursement system may lead to the closure of one out of every five existing hospitals during the first five years of the system's implementation.[11]

Beyond the satisfaction of intellectual curiosity there is no need to pursue here all possible ways in which the health care system may respond to current and emerging financial pressures. The shape and direction of most institutional responses will lie well beyond the control of the individual supervisor or manager within the institution. Rather, the primary interest of this volume is the consideration of how the individual supervisor's work is affected and what the supervisor can do about mounting cost containment pressure.

HEALTH CARE COST CONTAINMENT IS HERE TO STAY

The United States health care environment has changed dramatically in two critical, interrelated dimensions: the imposition of financial limitations on the system, and the advent of open competition.

Financial Limitations

The amount of money devoted to health care is not being allowed to increase at a rate naturally determined by the perceived needs of the system itself. The rate of growth is being deliberately slowed by the external im-position of regulatory mechanisms intended to stem the rise in the nation's health care bill by forcing changes to occur within the system. Further in-sight into how this is occurring is provided in Chapter 3, Reimbursement for Nonfinancial Managers.

Competition

Once almost universally discouraged and even today denied by some as harmful to the provision of quality health care, open competition among health care providers is increasing and is likely to become intense for several years as the health care system adjusts to external financial pressures.

In addition to regulatory pressure, other signs suggest the growth of con-ditions favoring competition. For example, the country is headed into a period of oversupply of physicians. During the decade of the 1970s, the number of physicians in the United States increased by 41 percent, a rate of increase far outdistancing the growth of the general population,[12] leading to undeniable increases in the number of physicians relative to patients. The average available patients per physician dropped 21 percent from 1970 to 1983, and this ratio is expected to drop another 20 percent by 1990.[13]

Unused hospital capacity will become a more prominent factor as further alternatives to short-term hospitalization are vigorously pursued for the sake of institutional survival. Despite the previously noted decline in the number of hospitals, and despite occasional problems of geographic distribution of facilities, overall there is considerable unused capacity within the hospital system. The health care providers that remain viable in the long run will be those who are able to provide quality care at competitive prices.

IMPLICATIONS FOR THE SUPERVISOR

The hospital is in a unique position as a health care provider with a strong interest in maintaining the level of income necessary to provide its service and remain solvent and also as an employer having to pay an increasing health care bill for a number of employees. The cost of employee health care coverage is fully as significant a budget item for a hospital as it is for a manufacturing or commercial enterprise with an equivalent number of employees. However, the manufacturing or commercial enterprise's only in-terest, as far as health care is concerned, is to stop the growth in the amount paid for health care coverage. But the hospital is involved in a rather elemen-tary conflict, on the one hand feeling the need to stem the growth of the bill for employee health care coverage and on the other hand desiring to main-tain the growth in income perceived as required to maintain operations. Fortunately, addressing this basic conflict should ordinarily call for little involvement by the individual cost center supervisor.

Although the individual departmental or cost center supervisor is not really involved in global matters of health care finance or in adjusting to competitive forces, marketing health care services, and realigning the services of the organization, the supervisor nevertheless has an important role—perhaps the key role—in health care cost containment. Consider the impact of the organization's goals on the actions of the individual supervisor at the department or cost center level. Hospital costs are distributed among various components approximately as follows:

- wages and salaries — 50 percent;
- employee benefits — 8 percent;
- contracted services — 7 percent;
- professional fees — 6 percent;
- capital expenditures — 6 percent;
- fuel and utilities — 6 percent;
- drugs and pharmaceuticals — 5 percent;
- food — 4 percent;
- medical supplies — 3 percent;
- all other expenses — 5 percent.[14]

Although a few of these cost elements lie largely or perhaps completely beyond the individual supervisor's control, at the department or cost center level most of these costs can be controlled or at least influenced through the actions of the supervisor. Thus the institution's success at controlling costs will be largely the sum of the successful efforts of individual supervisors. The most effective control is that exercised at the point in the organization where resources are actually applied.

The pass-through concept of pricing health care services (that is, the cost-plus approach, calling for all actual costs of providing service, plus a markup for profit, surplus, or coverage of bad debts or other items, to be passed directly through to the ultimate payer who then pays without question) is largely a practice of the past. Certainly it has always been the function of the health care supervisor to assure the delivery of quality patient care. It is now the function of the health care supervisor, and is likely to be for the foreseeable future, to assure the delivery of this quality care in a cost-effective manner.

It has long been the attitude of many working in health care that control of costs automatically leads to diminution of quality, that it is not possible to focus seriously on cost control and productivity improvement without impairing the organization's ability to sustain high quality. However, this attitude appears to be based on two implicit and generally fallacious assumptions: that there is a direct relationship between quality and cost (lowest quality means lowest cost, higher quality means higher cost, highest quality means highest cost); and that the present way of doing things represents the highest quality available for the money (the belief that it is not possible to improve today's cost picture without adversely affecting quality, and that it is not possible to increase quality without increasing cost).

Regardless of some present beliefs relative to the quality-versus-cost issue, undeniable forces have entered the health care system:

- Health care costs are being capped and will not be allowed to grow unchecked.
- Competition will become a way of life in health care.
- Continued high quality care will be demanded despite pressures to contain costs.

As has happened over the years in many industries other than health care, the control of costs and the enhancement of productivity will henceforth be critical elements of every supervisor's job.

NOTES

1. U.S. Bureau of the Census, *Statistical Abstract* (Washington, D.C.: GPO, 1960-1980).
2. R.M. Gibson and D.R. Waldo, "National Health Expenditures," *Health Care Financing Review*, September 1981.
3. Bureau of National Affairs, "Business, Labor Search for Solutions to Spiraling Health Care Expense," *White Collar Report* 54 (1983): 558.
4. *Resource*, February 1984, p. 2.
5. Cathy Schoen, "Maintaining and Improving Health Benefits by Containing Costs," *White Collar Report* 54 (1983): 535.
6. Ibid.
7. Bureau of National Affairs, "SEIU Plan to Press for Legislation on Cost Containment," *White Collar Report* 54 (1983): 518-519.
8. Ibid.
9. Gibson and Waldo, "National Health Expenditures."
10. U.S. National Center for Health Statistics, *Health Resources Statistics* (Washington, D.C.: GPO, 1968-1979).
11. Donald F. Beck, "The Hospital's Financial Future: DRGs and Beyond," *Health Care Supervisor* 3, no. 2 (January 1985): 5.
12. See note 10.
13. Schoen, "Maintaining and Improving Health Benefits by Containing Costs," p. 536.
14. Kenneth A. Johnson and Clifford Neely, "Hospital Economic Forecast," *Hospitals*, October 1, 1983, p. 87.

Part II

Budgeting and Control: How To Understand Bottom Lines and Work with Budgets without Being an Accountant

Chapter 2

The Basic Basics of Accounting

In an ordinary economic sense, all management people are "partners" and, as such, have a major stake in one another's achievements.

Robert Townsend

Chapter Objectives

- Define the basic accounting elements and processes.
- Review the more common financial reports and provide the supervisor with a starting point for learning to analyze and interpret these reports.
- Provide the supervisor who does not have a formal accounting background with a basic understanding of accounting processes.

ACCOUNTING IN PERSPECTIVE

Accounting may be broadly defined as a *systematic means of providing information on the economic affairs of an organization.*[1] Accounting provides much information for making business decisions. Directly and indirectly, managers and many others within an organzation regularly use the output of accounting processes. It is difficult to imagine how the complex economic structures of most modern organizations could operate without the information provided by extensive networks of accounting activities.

Considered in its entirety, accounting is a relatively complex business science. However, one need not be steeped in technical details of accounting to be able to grasp its principles. This chapter will lay the groundwork for the supervisor's understanding of a few simple but essential principles of accounting for the operation of a business organization. There is no need for the supervisor (except the supervisor of the accounting department) to be an accountant. But the supervisor must:

- know how to read and interpret simple financial statements;
- understand the common uses of certain finance terms;
- understand the general processes by which the institution is reimbursed for providing service;
- know how to develop and work with a budget.

Accounting

Bookkeeping may be described as the recording portion of accounting. That is, accounting consists of bookkeeping activities to which activities of summary and analysis have been added. Buried within the seeming complexities of accounting is simple double-entry bookkeeping, based on the principle of balance. As applied in double-entry bookkeeping, the principle of balance dictates that there be at least two entries made for every transaction so that entries can be checked against each other for verification.

Accounting Elements

All business transactions have effects on the basic accounting elements. These accounting elements are:

- assets, or that which is owned;
- liabilities, or that which is owed;
- equity, or the excess of assets over liabilities.

To identify further the accounting elements:

Assets:

An asset is anything that either exists as money or has some dollar value. The more common assets of an organization usually include cash, accounts receivable, land, buildings, equipment and furnishings, supplies on hand, and the like.

Liabilities:

A liability is anything that represents money owed to other organizations or persons. Common liabilities include accounts payable (money owed to suppliers), wages payable (money owed to employees), taxes payable (money owed to the government), loans and mortgages, and such.

Equity:

Equity is how much the enterprise is truly "worth" in terms of the excess of value owned (assets) over value of all outstanding obligations (liabilities). With regard to either an organization or an individual in business, equity may also be referred to by a number of other common terms including: *net worth, proprietorship*, and *capital*.

The Accounting Equation

The fundamental mathematical relationship underlying most accounting practice is simply:

$$\text{Assets} = \text{Liabilities} + \text{Equity}$$

Knowing any two elements of the equation, one can always determine the third element. Consider as a simple illustration the example of Mr. Smith, who owns a mortgaged house, is paying for an automobile over a period of three or four years, owns some household furnishings, has some money in the bank, and also has debts on a few accounts. Mr. Smith's assets might be:

Cash (in bank)	$ 2,000
Home	50,000
Furnishings	8,000
Automobile	6,000
Total Assets	$ 66,000

His liabilities appear as:

Unpaid bills	$ 1,000
Mortgage balance	42,000
Automobile loan	3,000
Total Liabilities	$ 46,000

Since Assets = Liabilities + Equity, then Equity = Assets − Liabilities. For Mr. Smith: Equity = $66,000 − $46,000, or Equity = $20,000. Thus Mr. Smith is "worth" $20,000 when one considers the excess value of everything he owns over the value of everything he owes.

Although the basic accounting equation is disarmingly simple in concept, the continuing application of the equation in actual practice can become extremely complex. One is required to keep track of constant change in the accounting elements. Every transaction that occurs directly alters one of the elements and can in turn affect one or both of the remaining elements. The problem is one of volume; even an enterprise that may be safely described as a small business may book hundreds of transactions in a day, and a moderately complex entity such as a full-service hospital may book thousands of transactions on an average business day. For every transaction it is necessary to capture the effects on one or more of the three basic accounting elements: assets, liabilities, and equity.

Debits and Credits

One ordinarily approaches accounting entries for the first time through consideration of the simple T-account (see Figure 2-1). Entries made to the left side of the T-account are called *debits*; entries made to the right side are called *credits*.

In considering debits and credits one must dispel the possibly held notion that some of these entries are "bad" and others are "good," or that these

---

Figure 2-1 The Simple T-Account

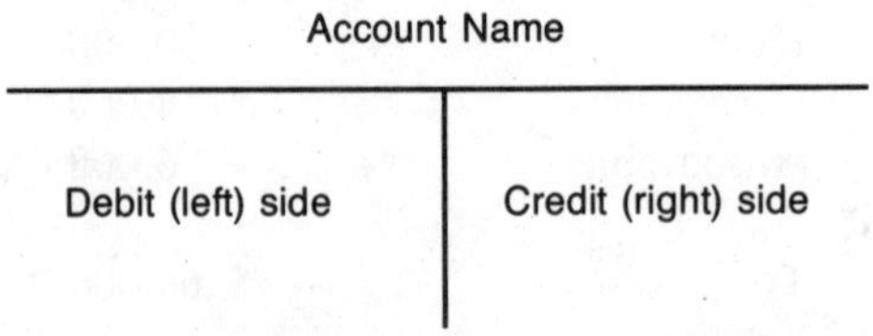

Account Name

Debit (left) side	Credit (right) side

entries invariably mean "in" or "out." Rather, these terms are simply accounting conventions consistent within a single dimension—a debit entry is always at the left side of an account, and a credit is always at the right side.

As to what debit and credit really mean, one needs to know what kind of account is involved, that is, which of the basic accounting elements is affected. Figure 2-2 displays the effects of debits and credits on the basic types of accounts.

Probably the easiest way to remember the impact of debits and credits is to relate their placement in the T-accounts to their effects on the basic accounting equation. The accounting equation is a true equation mathematically; that is, equality must always be preserved. Whenever one side of the equation is increased or decreased, the other side must be increased or decreased by an equal amount.

Consider a simple example in which a hospital receives a gift of a parcel of land valued at $10,000. Common sense suggests that this gift increases assets by $10,000, and that, since nothing is owed as a result of this transaction, equity is also increased by $10,000. In the basic accounting equation:

$$\text{Assets} = \text{Liabilities} + \text{Equity}$$

the impact of this single transaction is:

$$\text{Assets} + \$10,000 = \text{Liabilities} + (\text{Equity} + \$10,000)$$

Thus both the right and left sides of the equation have increased by $10,000 and the basic equality has been preserved. In this case the net increase in assets is reflected in a net increase in equity.

Figure 2-2 Effects of Debits and Credits

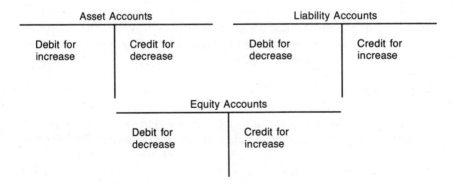

Generally T-accounts no longer exist in that particular form (the physical T-account, on paper) except in the smallest of enterprises (a few sole proprietors experiencing few transactions may still keep their books in this manner). However, the impact of debits and credits remains the same regardless of the relative sophistication of a given accounting system:

Debits always:
- increase assets;
- decrease liabilities;
- decrease equity.

Credits always:
- decrease assets;
- increase liabilities;
- increase equity.

At all times and for all transactions there is equal impact on the two sides of the basic accounting equation, so the principle of balance is preserved.

In most business organizations, what once was a collection of T-accounts on paper is presently a collection of data retained on magnetic tape or disk or stored in computer memory. Periodically (perhaps each day, perhaps only once in a while, depending on the accounts involved) this information is printed out in detail. As previously suggested, most problems that are encountered relate not to processes, which are relatively simple, but rather to sheer volume of information. An organization of any appreciable size may experience thousands of transactions each day affecting hundreds of accounts and subaccounts.

BASIC FINANCIAL REPORTS

The supervisor is quite regularly exposed to certain financial reports—collections of accounting data presented in specific ways intended to convey certain kinds of information. A few basic reports constitute most of the supervisor's exposure to financial statements.

Trial Balance

The trial balance is more of a process or working tool than a report. It is created periodically to prove that the accounts are in balance, that all debits do equal all credits. Since many transactions are likely to occur in a sizeable organization, there is a significant chance of occasional errors in posting to the numerous accounts. The trial balance may not initially be in balance; it then serves as a starting point for locating errors. Once the trial balance is brought into balance, the data can be used for subsequent reporting purposes.

Balance Sheet

The balance sheet is a financial statement summarizing all assets, liabilities, and equities in a manner that demonstrates the equality of the basic accounting equation. Certainly the most common and perhaps the most important financial statement in information provided, the balance sheet encapsulates the financial status of the enterprise for a given period and often compares multiple periods with each other. Table 2-1 shows a simplified balance sheet

Table 2-1 General Hospital Comparative Balance Sheet
December 31, 1984 (thousands of dollars)

	1984	1983	1982
Assets			
Cash	$ 12	$ (3)*	$ 51
Investments	215	78	12
Accounts Receivable	3,556	2,957	2,652
Inventories	487	404	472
Total Current Assets	4,270	3,436	3,187
Land	403	398	398
Buildings and Equipment	11,089	10,656	9,125
Total Assets	$ 15,762	$ 14,490	$ 12,710
Liabilities			
Accounts Payable	$ 687	$ 650	$ 642
Accrued Expenses	1,358	1,010	1,259
Notes Payable	222	163	163
Total Current Liabilities	2,267	1,823	2,064
Bonds Payable	2,326	2,511	710
Total Liabilities	$ 4,593	$ 4,334	$ 2,774
Equity			
Net Worth	$ 11,169	$ 10,156	$ 9,936
Liabilities plus Equity	$ 15,762	$ 14,490	$ 12,710

*( ) denotes a deficit

for a hypothetical hospital. This is referred to as a *comparative balance sheet* because it compares the results of 1984 with the results of previous years.

Note initially that the sum of equity and liabilities is equal to total assets, satisfying the basic accounting equation. Note also that equity (that is, what is owned minus what is owed) represents the true net worth of the hospital.

Table 2-1 introduces the use of the term *current* in reference to assets and liabilities. Assets are ordinarily listed on a balance sheet in approximate order of liquidity, that is, the ease with which they may be converted into cash. Current assets are those that exist as cash, are readily convertible to cash (such as accounts receivable), or are regularly turned over or consumed in the course of doing business.

Fixed assets, on the other hand, are assets that are not rapidly turned over, are not readily consumed, or are not readily convertible into cash. Most major fixed assets are comprised of land and depreciable items such as buildings and equipment.

Liabilities are usually likewise separated according to current, short-term obligations (those that must be satisfied out of current earnings) and long-term debt such as mortgages and bonds payable.

Balance sheets are often comparative. For example, Table 2-1 shows summarized results for 1984, 1983, and 1982. Note that net worth increased from 1982 to 1983 and again from 1983 to 1984. This indicates a profitable operation; had there been a loss, net worth would have shown a decrease from one year to the next.

Income Statement

The income statement, which may also be called a *profit and loss statement*, is a representation of performance of the enterprise from the end of one balance sheet period to the next.

Table 2-2 represents a simple income statement relating to the change in net worth from the end of 1983 to the end of 1984 on the balance sheet of Table 2-1. Net worth at the end of 1984 was $11,169,000; at the end of 1983 net worth was $10,156,000. The difference, $1,013,000, is the surplus—and thus an increase in net worth—generated by operations during 1984.

The income statement simply shows how the enterprise moved from one set of balance sheet results to the next. The balance sheet is a permanent record; the income statement, covering a single period, is temporary. Income statement accounts are temporary accounts in which information is collected until a convenient time for a summary to be generated. Practically speaking, equity remains frozen for a year at a time; during that year any transaction that would affect equity is recorded in an income statement account.

Table 2-2 General Hospital Income Statement, 1984

Income

Patient Revenues	$ 42,304,625	
Grants	425,000	
Miscellaneous Income	126,500	
Total Income		$ 42,856,126

Expenses

Wages and Salaries	22,460,925	
Employee Benefits	4,042,967	
Supplies and Other	13,824,381	
Depreciation	798,132	
Interest	356,720	
Total Expenses		$ 41,843,125
Net Operating Income		$ 1,013,000

At the end of the accounting year the income statement accounts are emptied (that is, the books are closed) and equity is changed to reflect either a gain or a loss on the balance sheet.

THE BASIC ACCOUNTING PROCESS, SIMPLIFIED

Initially a *chart of accounts* is established out of a determination of what accounts are required and how they should be numbered or otherwise identified.

As transactions occur, they are analyzed for their effects on the accounting elements. The first record created is a *journal* which captures at a minimum for each transaction:

- a description of the transaction;
- the date of the transaction;
- the amount of the transaction;
- the accounts affected and the appropriate amounts (balancing debits and credits).

Since the journal is chronological, an additional record is needed to provide the summary status of each account. This record is called the *ledger*, simply a grouping of accounts similar in character and arranged according to the accounting elements. Although there are only three types of accounts—asset accounts, liability accounts, and equity accounts—there may be many subgroups within each type and thus there may be many accounts within a ledger.

Periodically the books are closed (all transactions that apply to the period are entered) and a trial balance is run to verify the accuracy of the processes. When the trial balance has been proven, income statements and balance sheets are prepared as necessary.

COMPLICATING THE PROCESS

Although accounting is simple in basic theory, it can be complex in practice. It is complicated by the volume and wide variety of transactions, and it is especially complicated by problems of valuation.

Problems of valuation are addressed—and legal requirements are satisfied—by the adoption and application of a set of *generally accepted accounting principles* (GAAP).

Since balance sheets consist of numbers they may seem at times to be precise and factual, cut and dried. Every balance sheet item, it seems, has a distinct dollar value. However, it is necessary to question most balance sheet values and look beyond the dollar signs.

The balance sheet is supposed to capture the economic worth of the enterprise. However, the most it captures is a best guess of economic worth. Most balance sheet figures are estimates of one sort or another; often the only balance sheet asset that is not an estimate is cash.

A consistent approach to the valuation of worth is required. Thus a set of GAAP is needed. A common set of principles dictates that:

- Investments are valued at what the institution paid for them (although their value at the moment could be considerably higher or lower because of market performance).
- Accounts receivable are recorded net of an estimated allowance for bad debts.
- Land, buildings, and other fixed assets are valued at cost regardless of what their present market value may be.
- Equipment is valued according to what it cost, although it may be costlier to replace at present prices.

How the foregoing and other valuation tasks are handled from statement to statement is expressed in the institution's set of GAAP. These principles cannot—indeed they need not—represent actual, factual truth. Rather, they represent consistency. Statements portraying the change in the state of the enterprise will forever remain estimates, but with the consistency of estimating represented by a set of GAAP the change in the status of the enterprise from statement to statement can be determined with considerable accuracy. Although GAAP are only assumptions, they work because they are reasonable and especially because they are consistently applied.

QUICK ASSESSMENTS OF FINANCIAL HEALTH

Just as a patient's vital signs—temperature, pulse, and respiration—can provide indications of the state of health, a number of signs can be read quickly for some indication of the financial health of an enterprise. Like human vital signs, however, there is a range of acceptable results, and variations do not always mean problems. It is a mistake to read too much into any particular indicator; nevertheless the use of quick indicators can be helpful in understanding the state of the organization.

The several indicators discussed are presented with examples derived from Table 2-3, a comparative balance sheet for a hypothetical hospital. All examples use the figures from the 1984 column of Table 2-3.

Current Ratio

The current ratio is simply the ratio of current assets to current liabilities:

$$\frac{\text{Current Assets}}{\text{Current Liabilities}} = \frac{\$8,401.4}{\$3,102.3} = 2.71 \text{ to } 1$$

This crude measure is commonly used to assess the ability of an enterprise to meet all of its current obligations with some margin of safety. A current ratio in the range of 2 to 1 may be considered risky (and less than 1 to 1 indicates insolvency). A current ratio greater than 3 to 1 is healthy but not necessarily desirable; it can suggest that too much money may be in the form of idle cash or that too much money may be tied up in inventories.

Liquidity Ratio

The liquidity ratio is:

$$\frac{\text{Cash} + \text{Short-term Investments} + \text{Accounts Receivable}}{\text{Current Liabilities}}$$

$$\text{or } \frac{\$3,926.7 + \$1,981.6 + \$2,001.3}{\$3,102.3} = 2.55 \text{ to } 1$$

Table 2-3 Community Hospital Comparative Balance Sheet
December 31, 1984 (thousands of dollars)

Assets	1984	1983
Cash	$ 3,926.7	$ 2,959.7
Short-term Investments	1,981.6	1,978.2
Accounts Receivable	2,001.3	2,153.6
Supplies Inventory	414.6	398.7
Prepaid Expenses	77.2	61.3
Total Current Assets	$ 8,401.4	$ 7,551.5
Land and Buildings	$ 11,421.6	$ 11,892.1
Equipment	9,815.4	10,015.0
Plant Replacement Fund	6,443.8	5,827.7
Long-term Investments	4,467.7	3,986.3
Total	$ 32,148.5	$ 31,721.1
Liabilities and Net Worth		
Accounts Payable	$ 620.9	$ 1,250.3
Accrued Expenses	1,729.1	1,388.2
Payroll Taxes and Deductions Payable	328.8	253.9
Long-term Debt, Current Year	425.5	420.2
Total Current Liabilities	$ 3,102.3	$ 3,312.6
Long-term Debt	$ 8,510.7	$ 8,403.0
Net Worth	20,535.5	20,005.5
Total Liabilities and Net Worth	$ 32,148.5	$ 31,721.1

Like the current ratio, this ratio also tests the organization's ability to meet short-term obligations. However, this is a harsher test because it concentrates on liquid assets of fairly certain value; eliminated in this example were supplies inventory and prepaid expenses, neither of which could probably be converted into their full cash value.

A liquidity ratio of at least 1 to 1 is desirable, which would indicate that if the organization closed its doors at this moment all of the bills could still be paid. Our example suggests that perhaps Community Hospital could safely shift some current assets into longer-term investments.

Debt-to-Assets Relationship

The debt-to-assets relationship is the percentage of total debt to total assets:

$$\frac{\text{Total Debt}}{\text{Total Assets}} (100) = \frac{\$3,102.3 + \$8,510.7}{\$32,148.5} (100) = 36.1 \text{ percent}$$

This equation provides a quick indication of how much of the enterprise is being run on borrowed money. The lower this percentage, the larger the financial cushion available to absorb possible losses.

Accounts Receivable Turnover

Accounts receivable turnover can be explained as follows: Assume that Community Hospital received patient revenues totaling $10,439,000 for 1984 and that revenues are continuing at the same average rate, which is $28,600 per day (not shown in Table 2-3 but in Community Hospital's income statement).
Then:

$$\frac{\text{Accounts Receivable}}{\text{Revenue per day}} = \frac{\$2,001,300}{\$28,600} = 70 \text{ days}$$

Thus the hospital has an average of 70 days' billings tied up in accounts receivable. A high number of days signals that steps should be considered to reduce the accounts receivable. Indeed, the higher this number the more worthwhile it is to bring it down. In the example, bringing outstanding receivables down from 70 days to 50 days would increase the hospital's cash position by $572,000. If the annual interest rate of 12 percent is the value of money, 20 days' interest on the reduction in receivables amounts to $3,761. Since receivables have to be financed either by borrowed money or by money that could otherwise be used elsewhere, reducing outstanding receivables produces tangible savings.

An Exercise

As a simple exercise, it is suggested that the reader use the 1983 column of Table 2-3 and calculate all of the foregoing ratios and percentages for that year and decide whether there is a basis for any tentative conclusions concerning the relative financial stability of Community Hospital.

WORKING FAMILIARITY

There is no requirement that the health care supervisor be an accountant. However, neither should the supervisor regard finance as entirely foreign. Every health care supervisor should have a working familiarity with basic accounting concepts and terms; the job demands such if it is to be done well. Ideally the supervisor should:

- understand basic accounting elements: assets, liabilities, and equity;
- understand the effects of debits and credits on accounting elements;
- know the basic financial reports, i.e., what they are and what information they are intended to convey.

The conscientious supervisor can benefit from self-guided practice in reading, interpreting, and analyzing financial reports and asking questions about what is not understood. An active interest in the financial status of the institution will likely increase the supervisor's value and effectiveness and will enable him or her to provide more informed and thus more effective cost control.

NOTE

1. Myron J. Gordon and Gordon Shillinglaw, *Accounting: A Management Approach*, 3rd ed. (Homewood, Ill.: Richard D. Irwin, 1964), p. 3.

Chapter 3

Reimbursement for Nonfinancial Managers

Eloquence avails nothing against the voice of gold.

Latin Proverb

Chapter Objectives

- Present an overview of the rise and spread of reimbursement regulation in the health care industry.
- Develop a general concept of reimbursement rate setting as applied by the major third party payers.
- Outline the general processes involved in the new federal prospective payment system for Medicare and examine the implications of this approach.
- Examine the effects of reimbursement regulation on management decision making in the health care environment.

THE RISE OF REGULATION

In nonregulated business there are a producer and a consumer. The producer offers a product or a service and sets the price for it according to fixed and variable costs, desired profit margins, and market forces. The consumer orders the product or service and pays for it at the going price.

Two critical factors make health care dramatically different from a nonregulated business:

1. In health care the service is ordinarily not ordered directly by the consumer (patient). Ordering is done by a physician, a representative and advisor of the consumer.
2. Neither the consumer nor the consumer's representative pays the producer. The producer or provider of health care service is paid, for the most part, by third parties.

In the context of health care reimbursement a third party payer is simply one that pays for service on behalf of an individual who is either insured by the third party or who subscribes to a program offered by the third party. The major third party payers in the country are Blue Cross and Blue Shield, nonprofit health insurance companies, and Medicare and Medicaid, which are government programs. Also, commercial insurance companies that deal in health insurance are third party payers.

Third party payers' funds come from premiums paid directly by individuals, premiums paid by employer organizations on behalf of employees, taxes paid to state and federal governments, and in some cases combinations of these. Funds of Blue Cross and Blue Shield come from individual and employer premiums; Medicaid's funds come largely from various taxes; Medicare's money comes chiefly from taxes supplemented by individuals' premiums for certain kinds of coverage. Although certain forms of health insurance have been available in the United States since the middle 1800s, health insurance did not begin to be widespread until after the establishment of Blue Cross in 1937.

The first active government involvement in health care regulation came from the Hill-Burton Act of 1946, which provided construction funds for health care facilities. Along with Hill-Burton came health facility accountability for the use of funds so acquired, and requirements for charity care to be provided by institutions accepting Hill-Burton money in annual amounts related to their Hill-Burton grants.

Prior to 1966, Blue Cross and commercial insurers provided health insurance coverage for the largest share of the United States population. These insurers simply paid billed charges, as did a lesser but still significant number of patients who had no insurance coverage and thus paid their own bills. In 1965, however, the stage was set for permanent and ultimately drastic change in the way the nation paid its hospital bills when the federal Medicare and Medicaid programs—Title XVII and Title XVIII of the Social Security Act—were signed into law by President Lyndon B. Johnson.

Medicare began on July 1, 1966, as a national program administered by the federal government through a network of intermediaries, primarily the country's various Blue Cross plans. Medicare was intended as insurance primarily for those aged 65 and older, and it was established to pay amounts not based on charges of health care providers but rather on reasonable costs of providing service.

Medicaid, although also a national program, was established for administration by the states, with some federal reimbursement, in compliance with various federal requirements. Since the beginning of Medicaid the states have differed in their eligibility requirements for Medicaid and in the variety of services provided under individual programs.

Although many measures were debated and proposed in the halls of government during the 1970s and early 1980s, the next major change in the federal government's role in health care payment did not occur until the passage of the Omnibus Budget Reconciliation Act of 1981. This act required significant reductions in federal health care expenditures, increased Medicare deductibles, and development of a prospective reimbursement methodology (that is, a system in which the exact payment for any particular service would be specified in advance).

In 1982, the Tax Equity and Fiscal Responsibility Act (TEFRA) included changes intended to reduce federal expenditures for Medicare. The federal government had by now made plain that it would be intimately involved in the regulation of health care reimbursement.

While the federal government was pondering and proposing, various individual states were becoming increasingly active in reimbursement regulation. Progress in reimbursement regulation overall, however, was difficult to measure because regulation through the 1970s was in the hands of the states and the states did not proceed in parallel with each other. Some states were highly restrictive while others were flexible in their regard for health care reimbursement.

Because the individual states reacted differently during the 1970s to the increasing financial pressure caused by rising health care costs, by 1982:

- about 20 percent of states had moved to restrict the number of days of care that would be paid for or the length of stay that would be approved for any particular diagnosis requiring hospital inpatient care;

- 25 to 30 percent of states had reduced the scope of reimbursable services or had eliminated reimbursement for some services entirely;
- about 20 percent of states had altered their payment guidelines to eliminate inappropriate use of emergency rooms and outpatient services;
- about 40 percent of states had restricted or reduced hospital inpatient reimbursement overall, including 13 states that had introduced forms of intended prospective payment;
- 30 percent of states had introduced requirements for prior authorization for the use of various services and requirements for second opinions for elective surgery;
- 30 percent of states had increased third party liability for recovery efforts (aimed at retrieving overpayments and inappropriate payments from providers).

Also by 1982, 20 percent of the states had expanded Medicaid eligibility and 25 percent had added reimbursement for new services (although some of these new services were intended to avoid costlier hospitalization and thus save money generally).

Three states have had several years' experience with statewide, all-payer reimbursement: Massachusetts, New Jersey, and New York. Since statewide reimbursement regulation has been pursued for the greatest length of time in New York, it will be useful to review briefly the experience of that state.

THE NEW YORK EXPERIENCE

Concerned with increases in Medicaid costs from 1966 to 1969, New York passed its cost control legislation in 1969. Effective January 1, 1970, this legislation:

1. required that the rates paid to hospitals for providing care no longer be based on "reasonable cost" as had been the case previously, but would henceforth be based on the cost of "the efficient production of hospital services."
2. gave New York the authority to regulate the rates paid by Blue Cross, effectively coupling Blue Cross and Medicaid.

With its cost control legislation of 1969, New York took the first major step toward leading the country into the era of widespread financial regulation of health care. Coupling Blue Cross with Medicaid allowed New York to control approximately half of all hospital revenue by legally forcing institutions to comply with cost control regulations.

Despite the label of cost control, however, the major impact of New York regulations had been revenue control. By limiting revenues, the state forced costs into line. From the beginning of 1970 to the end of 1975, New York controls helped to stimulate a significant reduction in the rate of increase of health care costs in the state. There was also another major force that helped moderate the rate of growth of health care costs in New York and the nation as a whole during this same period—the Economic Stabilization Program in effect from August 14, 1971, to April 30, 1974. The Economic Stabilization Program, widely referred to as the "wage-price freeze," imposed generally more rigid controls on health care than on other industries.

Mounting financial problems in New York and its major cities led to severe cutbacks, effective January 1, 1976, in the amount of Medicaid reimbursement paid to health care institutions. The state's reimbursement formula was tightened and allowable costs were further restricted. Because of the legal coupling of major health insurance programs the cutbacks applied to Blue Cross as well, so the total effect on institutions was relatively severe.

In 1978, the New York State Office of Health Systems Management (OHSM), an arm of the state's Department of Health, was given the power to control inpatient hospital charges. Thus the state consolidated its control of inpatient payments to hospitals by Medicaid, Workers' Compensation, No-Fault Insurance, Blue Cross, commercial insurance carriers, and private payers. The only remaining exclusion from state control was federal Medicare. Finally, in 1983, Medicare in New York was brought under state control, which gave the state complete control over inpatient reimbursement.

The theory of New York's control has always proclaimed the basis of limiting payment to the cost of the efficient delivery of service. In practice, however, more often than not payment has been capped by the state's total budgetary limitations. This reimbursement philosophy has been seen by many as leading more than a few health care institutions into substantial deficits, and has supposedly forced some institutions into bankruptcy and encouraged others to seek mergers and other affiliations. And this comprehensive, highly regulatory approach to health care reimbursement has focused a great deal of hospital management attention on a single fundamental goal, staying in existence.

THE CONCEPT OF RATE SETTING

A general theory of rate setting can be inferred from the assumptions implicit in the behavior of third party payers, those insurers and government agencies that actually pay for health care service. The third party payers appear to assume that:

1. They cannot pay based solely on charges because charges may vary greatly among institutions and may also include substantial profit or surplus factors as well as charges that the payers cannot or will not support, such as bad debts, unneeded services, and personal preference items (such as telephones or televisions).
2. It is possible to develop rate formulas that will appropriately pay for care given to patients covered under each different payer's program.
3. A uniform reimbursement formula for all institutions will yield fair and consistent rates.
4. A formula that uses only known and approved elements of cost will assure payment only for services that the payers' programs are established to cover.

In practice, however, each payer develops its own payment methodology separately from all other payers. Each paying organization individually applies further assumptions about its own population, and often the combined effects of various payment methodologies can be negative. Medicare, for instance, assumes that its population requires on the average less daily inpatient service than the so-called usual "average" patient requires, and the Medicare methodology is structured to reflect this assumed difference. On the other hand, Medicaid and Blue Cross assume that their populations are truly average and thus use formulas based on average cost.

For illustration consider a situation in which a hospital receives revenues of 35 percent from Medicare, 50 percent from Medicaid and Blue Cross combined, and 15 percent from all other sources. Half of the hospital's reimbursement is based on average costs so it can expect to get back what it spent for Medicaid and Blue Cross patients. However, Medicare's 35 percent being reimbursed on less-than-average cost saddles the institution with a guaranteed shortfall on every patient making up part of the 35 percent. Together 85 percent of the hospital's patients are assumed to absorb average costs or less, but none of them are officially regarded as absorbing costs above the average. For years the practice was to attempt to make up the shortfall by applying higher charges to the remaining 15 percent of the patient population. However, in states subject to charge control it is no longer possible to continue raising charges for those payers outside of the Medicare-Medicaid-Blue Cross triad. Also, it is unrealistic to assume that the hospital's remaining 15 percent of patients can make up the difference because in addition to payments by commercial insurers and private payers, there are uninsured and charity care patients. Thus the concept of rate setting as applied in an expanding regulatory environment simply increases the chances that the individual institution will lose money.

DIAGNOSTIC RELATED GROUPS: TRUE PROSPECTIVITY ARRIVES

With the coming of TEFRA, on January 1, 1982, the federal government set targets for the maximum allowable annual increase in spending on behalf of patients covered by government programs. For 1982 the spending increase target was 7.2 percent. However, there were problems with target rates: these rates did not allow for differences in labor costs from region to region and did not allow for the inherently higher costs of teaching hospitals.

Within months of passage most parts of TEFRA dealing with spending for health care were displaced by prospective payment legislation. Prospective payment for hospitals was officially enacted in March 1983 under Title VI of the Social Security Amendments of 1983 (Public Law 98-21). This legislation mandated true prospective payment; that is, it required that the exact amounts hospitals would be receiving for providing service be known in advance.

The Medicare Bureau of the Health Care Financing Administration (HCFA) selected the diagnostic related group (DRG) system as its prospective payment mechanism. As the most dramatic change in third party payment ever attempted, payment for Medicare patients using rates established by DRGs entered its initial phase on January 1, 1984.

DRGs represent an effort to control costs by setting advance prices for service completely independent of any particular hospital's cost structure. Thus DRGs are seen by many as indicating the arrival of real prospectivity. Various state approaches had been labeled as "prospective" systems but in reality these were retrospective; even though providers may have received predetermined payments, these payments were subject to retroactive adjustments after the providers' costs were audited (often years after occurrence).

In establishing the basis for DRG reimbursement, the system's developers initially considered more than 10,000 possible illnesses and procedures and placed them in major diagnostic categories based on 23 body systems. So categorized, all of these illnesses and procedures were then reduced through extensive statistical analysis to 467 DRGs.

For every Medicare patient with any particular diagnosis or procedure, a given hospital will receive the same amount of money regardless of the patient's length of stay and regardless of services actually rendered. A hospital that spends more in providing care than the DRG pays must absorb the loss; a hospital that spends less than the DRG pays is allowed to keep the surplus.

DRG prices are intended to vary among geographic regions and among various hospitals within regions for at least three years. By the fourth year of the system it is intended that all hospitals in the country be reimbursed at the same average cost, that is, using a national DRG determined by the federal government. All DRGs are to be reviewed every four years to allow for cost increases that may have accrued as a result of changes in medical technology.

The DRG system is intended in part to shrink the hospital system at points of unused or underutilized capacity. Simply stated, with income strictly controlled a hospital cannot financially support programs, staff, or facilities that are not being used regularly and thus are not bringing in enough money to cover their costs.

The price paid for each of the 467 DRGs was developed as follows:

1. Using 1980 Medicare cost reports, the federal government developed a case mix index, a numerical representation of intensity of service, for every hospital.
2. In consideration of case mix, the 1980 cost per discharge was determined for each hospital.
3. Average costs per discharge were determined by state and by region according to hospital bed complement and other factors (such as, teaching or nonteaching).
4. The country was divided into eight geographic regions.
5. Each hospital in each region was put into one of two classes, rural or urban.
6. By region and by class of hospital, each DRG was priced using a grand average of 16 average costs per discharge.
7. Costs for 1980 were rolled into the following years using a predetermined hospital cost inflation factor.

To ease the impact of an inevitable dramatic change in Medicare reimbursement for many hospitals, the system is to be phased in over a three-year period. Thus any particular hospital would be reimbursed for its Medicare patients as follows:

First Year:
    25 percent by regional DRG
    75 percent cost-report based (under TEFRA)

Second Year:
    12.5 percent by national average DRG
    37.5 percent by regional DRG
    50 percent cost-report based

Third Year:
    37.5 percent by national average DRG
    37.5 percent by regional DRG
    25 percent cost-report based

Fourth and Subsequent Years:
    100 percent by national average DRG

It should be stressed that the foregoing is but a simplification of the highlights of the federal government's prospective reimbursement system. Details of the system—perhaps minor when the total system is considered, but significant to many individual institutions whose income depends on the system—are being debated at all levels of government and within all hospital forums and are being refined and altered almost daily.

The DRG reimbursement system may prove to be extremely complex. It will most certainly be complicated by the probability that many hospitals will appeal their case mix indexes, since these may have changed from 1980 to 1984. At least there will be appeals by hospitals whose case mix indexes appeared to have increased, that is, their levels of intensity have apparently increased. Many hospitals that have experienced reductions in levels of intensity may remain silent in hopes of protecting their reimbursement levels.

The long-run effects of reimbursement under the DRG approach are yet to be determined. However, there has been a great deal of doom-and-gloom forecasting regarding this dramatically different reimbursement approach. Under the prospective payment system a few hospitals that are presently strong financially may become stronger still as they "make money" from DRG reimbursement, but it is even more likely that many hospitals will suffer financially under DRGs.

Overall, the effects of the federal Medicare prospective payment system are likely to be:

- The federal government will save billions of dollars per year in what it pays for services to Medicare patients.
- Some hospitals will discontinue unused and underutilized services and specialize in the services that they can deliver profitably, that is, they will specialize in the services that are best economically.
- Some hospitals will merge with others or become part of existing multihospital chains, in search of management and scale economies that improve the chance of survival.
- Some hospitals will close their doors and leave the business of delivering inpatient care.

There will of course be no diminution in the general insistence from governments and individuals alike on high quality hospital care. In addition to all of the nonfinancial controls that exist to encourage efficient medical practice and the delivery of quality care, the DRG prospective payment system will strongly encourage efficient financial management of hospitals.

Given the pattern of major government change in regulatory directions, it is possible that the DRG approach may last only five to seven years before it is modified significantly or replaced with a different approach.[1]

MANAGEMENT DECISION MAKING UNDER REIMBURSE-MENT REGULATION

In a so-called normal business, meaning one that is not strictly regulated, expenses and revenues are independent of each other. Changing expenses will have no effect on the stream of revenue and changing prices (that is, varying revenue) will not affect expenses. The business always has the option of attempting to compensate for a projected loss by cutting costs or by increasing prices.

In health care institutions, however, normal business practices do not apply. Payers use institutions' costs to determine what revenues will be, so under many payment schemes changing expenses will therefore alter revenues. If a hospital that is projecting a loss cuts its costs, it also automatically reduces future revenues. In addition, the institution usually cannot change its revenues by raising prices because its revenues are determined by the payer independent of pricing.

Thus management decision making in health care institutions is made more complex by reimbursement regulations. Overall, reimbursement regulations have created a number of controversies and have given rise to a number of major reimbursement issues pertinent to the management of health care institutions.

Major Reimbursement Issues

The experiences of institutions in those geographic areas (primarily states) that have worked for several years under regulation have brought about the identification of issues, problems, concerns, and controversies including:

- Some reimbursement systems (the system of New York is a prime example) are so complex that they are not readily understood by those managers whose organizations' reimbursement depends on them.

Understanding these systems requires prolonged experience at studying and working with them, processes that frequently preclude management from making informed decisions. In some places it has become a virtual necessity to have full-time reimbursement specialists on staff.

- Within some systems, institutions may actually be penalized for saving money. Consider, for example, a hospital that has been effective in reducing length of stay through conscientious utilization review and efficient pre-admission testing and other processes. This hospital may be effective in reducing the total cost of a hospital stay, but because the stay is shorter the average cost of each day may be higher than before the cost-saving measures were applied so the hospital may be penalized because its per diem cost now exceeds "average."

- More and more health care money is seen as being spent on regulation and system administration, which does little or nothing to maintain or improve the quality of care available.

- Blue Cross and Medicaid assume that their patients are "average." Medicare assumes that its patients are something less than average in the care they require. Reimbursesment is determined on the basis of average cost or less but never on more than average cost, so institutions face built-in losses unless they are fortunate enough to have other sources that can make up the difference.

- Blue Cross and Medicaid rates are supposedly based on the cost of the efficient delivery of service. In practice, however, these rates are determined primarily by the money that can be made available in state budgets.

- A large number of patients, such as the working poor, illegal aliens, and others, are not covered by third party payers. Institutions are experiencing losses because the system forces these people into the private pay category without providing recourse for the bad debts inevitably experienced.

- Reimbursement appeal processes are generally cumbersome. An institution can require from several months to several years to obtain a justified rate adjustment.

- Retroactive adjustments can occur years after the time periods to which they apply.

Either singly or in some combination with each other, the foregoing issues and concerns affect management decision making in most of the country's health care institutions. Normally accepted cause-and-effect relationships are not present in the financial management of the health care delivery system, so an institution's management is expected to operate a business entity while being denied the ability to follow accepted business practice.

COSTS, REIMBURSEMENT, AND THE SUPERVISOR

Whether the DRG approach will take hold and eventually spread to cover total hospital reimbursement or will be replaced by a yet unknown reimbursement scheme remains to be seen. It is clear, however, that regardless of the specific approach followed, hospital costs will not be permitted to grow at the rates experienced in recent years. Not only will the rate of growth be moderated by such semi-artificial means, for some institutions it is even possible that absolute present dollar levels of reimbursement will be reduced.

The health care delivery environment will become increasingly competitive as institutions vie for patients and go head-to-head with each other on the basis of the cost-effective delivery of service. Almost every individual supervisor and manager in every institution will be brought under increasing pressure to reduce and hold down costs. There will be little choice in the matter; in many institutions, conscientious cost containment will be required for survival.

Even if DRGs and other present reimbursement mechanisms vanish within the coming several years, what remains in their place will sustain the pressure on costs. In all likelihood, health care cost regulation is permanent.

All supervisors' activities affect costs in some way. Some supervisors' activities directly affect reimbursement levels as well as costs. How well an institution performs financially is ultimately the sum of how well all of its supervisors and managers perform individually in regard to costs versus revenues.

Managers at all levels, and especially first-line supervisors with cost-center budget responsibility, are likely to discover in years to come that cost and cost-center financial performance will be among the most important criteria on which their performance is evaluated. Thus cost consciousness will be a necessity for every health care supervisor if he or she is to be fully effective.

NOTE
1. Donald F. Beck, "The Hospital's Financial Future: DRGs and Beyond," *Health Care Supervisor* 3, no. 2 (January 1985): 30.

Chapter 4

Building and Using a Budget*

Budgets must not be prepared on high and cast as pearls before swine.

Robert Townsend

Chapter Objectives

- Introduce the basic concepts of budgeting and establish the importance of budget preparation to the supervisor.
- Describe the advantages of participative approaches to budgeting.
- Define the various components of an institution's budget.
- Provide a step-by-step illustration of the preparation of a departmental budget.
- Describe the process of developing an institution's annual budget from the budgets of individual departments.
- Illustrate the fundamentals of the process of monitoring expenditures against budget allocations.

---

*Portions of this chapter were adapted from Charles R. McConnell, *The Effective Health Care Supervisor* (Rockville, Md.: Aspen Systems Corp., 1982), pp. 217–234.

INTRODUCING THE BUDGET

There are likely to be considerable differences in the ways different supervisors approach the contents of this chapter. In some health care institutions, individual supervisors have been actively involved in the budgeting process for years. In other institutions, however, the budget remains a mysterious collection of numbers assembled by the finance office with no direct supervisory involvement whatsoever.

One who has often been directly involved in the preparation of department budgets will find little in this chapter that has not been encountered in practice. If one's budget preparation experience is minimal or nonexistent, however, some assistance will be offered by this elementary view of budgeting. This chapter provides an overview of the budget and budgeting process and offers some specifics in a manner intended for consideration by supervisors who do not have backgrounds in accounting and finance (the vast majority of supervisors).

A budget is a financial plan that serves as an estimate of future operations and, to some extent, as a means of control over those operations. It is a quantitative statement of the organization's expressed operating intentions, and it translates these intentions into numbers and dollar signs.

A budget can be several things to the organization and to the individual supervisor. Used as a control mechanism, it can be a cost containment tool that helps keep costs in line with available resources. It can also be a basis for performance evaluation, since performance against a budget provides an indication of how well one utilizes the resources under one's control. Further, a budget can be a means for directing efforts toward productivity improvement—since performance against budget, in revealing how well resources are utilized, can give the supervisor a basis from which to work for improved utilization.

Participative Budgeting

In some hospitals and other health care organizations the budget is still prepared "upstairs" and handed down for supervisors and department heads to live with. This practice leaves much to be desired, since it requires the supervisor to implement a plan without having participated in that plan's development. The supervisor may remain ignorant of many of the whys and wherefores of the budget and thus be in a position of weakness when it comes to translating the department's financial plan into action.

Fortunately, however, more and more health care institutions are bringing their supervisors into the budgeting process. The team approach to budgeting, requiring active participation of managers at all levels, calls for close coordination of many diverse inputs and activities. It takes considerably more time and effort to assemble a budget in this manner than it does simply to allow administration and finance to work together and issue a budget, but the results of the team approach are usually worth the extra work. The participative approach to budgeting has several distinct advantages:

- The end item of the process, the budget, is usually a more realistic and workable plan than any that could be developed by some other means.
- The involvement of individual supervisors in the process breeds their commitment; they are more likely to believe in the budget and strive to make it work because they have taken part in its development.
- The interdepartmental and intradepartmental activities and interpersonal contacts pursued during the process tend to strengthen supervisors in their jobs.
- A spirit and an attitude of teamwork are created in getting managers at all levels to work together toward a common goal. Teamwork is, to a great extent, one of the keys to successful operation of an organization.
- The encouragement of more realistic planning serves to sharpen the focus of management's efforts and produce more appropriate results more often.

The involvement of the individual supervisor in the creation of the budget helps to define clearly the authority the supervisor possesses and the responsiblity with which that key person is charged in the operation of the department. Quite simply, you created your budget, so you are responsible for operating on that budget.

Although the responsibility for draft budget preparation may lie with the supervisor, there is no reason for involvement not to extend below that level. As portions of this chapter will reveal, there are certain budget-related activities (such as the accumulation of operating statistics) in which some of the department's employees could participate. Employees who understand the nature of the budget and the reasons behind its preparation are more likely to share actively in the objectives of the department.

Accounting Concepts

Before entering into a discussion of how a budget is structured, explanations of a pair of simple but important accounting concepts are in order: the fiscal year and fixed-versus-flexible budgets.

The fiscal year is simply the organization's 12-month accounting year. This may be any consecutive 12-month period established for accounting purposes; for instance, May 1 of this year to April 30 of next year; this means that for accounting purposes the institution's year begins on May 1. However, the fiscal year is just as likely to coincide with the calendar year beginning January 1. Through the decade of the 1970s the governments of numerous states encouraged health care institutions to use the calendar year as their fiscal year if they were not already doing. so. Also, increasing activity leading toward uniform accounting and reporting for health care institutions will probably result in the eventual adoption of the calendar fiscal year by all health care provider organizations.

Within the accounting year are a number of accounting periods. It is common practice to keep track of payroll and certain other expenses on the basis of one, two, or four weeks and to accumulate this information on the basis of the four-week accounting period. Thus there are 13 such accounting periods in the year. Other important facts and figures are accumulated by month, however, either because it is necessary to do so or because this is the best data collection period available. Accountants and others speak of the monthly closing, the act of determining the financial results of operations for a given month.

One of the biggest troubles encountered in budgeting involves differences in the length of the periods for which some data are accumulated. As noted, payroll data are almost always kept in two- or four-week periods; many other expenses and various operating statistics are accumulated by the month. In developing a budget, and especially in examining the results of operations after the fact, it is frequently necessary to manipulate some of the figures by adding in or taking out certain numbers at either end of the given period so one can develop complete information for the period of interest.

The concepts of fixed and flexible budgeting refer to the structural character of the budget relative to activity throughout the year. A fixed budget, by far the simpler of the two, assumes a stable level of operations throughout the year and spreads all budgeted costs evenly across the 12 months. A flexible budget, however, recognizes that certain costs can vary as the level of operations varies and attempts to account for this variation in the budget. A flexible budget may treat certain costs as fixed because they are in fact fixed or because this is simply the best way to handle them, but it will also attempt to identify and allow for costs that vary as department activity varies.

THE TOTAL BUDGET

There are several parts to the institution's overall budget, some calling for the supervisor's involvement and some that the supervisor will rarely be concerned with. The parts and subparts of the total budget described in the following sections are each thoroughly identified as budgets in their own right. If we seem to be saying "A budget is a part of a budget," we do so in the sense in which these financial plans have always been described.

The Operating Budget

The operating budget usually consists of three parts, the statistical, the expense, and the revenue budgets.

Statistical Budget:

The statistical budget is made up of projections of activity for the coming budget year. Usually based on a combination of past activity, current trends, and some limited knowledge of future conditions and circumstances, this is the organization's best estimate of work activity for the coming 12-month period. These estimates are projections of statistics, such as admissions or discharges expected, patient days expected, probable number of laboratory tests or x-ray procedures, number of meals to be served, pounds of linen to be processed, and so on. These may be prepared as gross, fixed estimates of the year's activity, or they may be projected by month based on certain knowledge suggesting variations in activity.

In getting ready to prepare the budget for the institution, the accounting department will generally compile and summarize the most recent historical data and projections available and supply this information to the other departments. It is often necessary, however, for departments to refine these figures into detailed estimates of activities for the coming budget year. The supervisor accomplishes this refinement the same way the accounting department makes its projections: based on past activity in the department and one's own knowledge of future operations.

Expense Budget:

The expense budget attempts to account for costs of operations (personnel and all other costs) for each department individually and for the institution as a whole. The departmental expense budget is the major area of supervisory involvement in the budgeting process. A simple step-by-step illustration of the preparation of a departmental expense budget is presented later in this chapter.

Revenue Budget:

Usually prepared by the accounting department, the revenue budget is a projection of the income likely to be received by the institution during the budget year. In view of the fact that revenue must ultimately cover all costs of operation, the revenue budget must attempt to consider the impact of numerous factors beyond the simple earning of income from services. A revenue budget may, for instance, attempt to reflect: the impact of a new service coming into being during the budget year; the effects of a service being deleted or curtailed during the year; additions to or departures from the medical staff that have bearing on number of admissions; the impact of decisions and recommendations of applicable health planning agencies; and the effects of changes in reimbursement regulations introduced by the major third party payers or by governments.

As noted earlier, the bulk of revenue of health care institutions comes from third party payers with some from patients themselves. There are also other sources of revenue that may include general donations, United Fund allocations, taxes (in the case of government institutions), research grants, investments, school operating revenues, television and telephone charges, purchase discounts, and cafeteria income.

Certain legitimate or potential deductions from revenue need to be considered as well. These include free care (hospitals are required to render such in certain amounts if they have accepted money under the federal Hill-Burton program), outright charity care, discounts to employees, and bad debts.

The Capital Budget

A capital budget is prepared to account for potential expenditures for major fixed and moveable equipment. Fixed equipment (a building, a boiler, or a new roof) and major moveable equipment (copy machines, hospital beds, x-ray machines, or computers) represent those costs that must be capitalized. These costs apply to operations for considerably longer than the coming budget period, so they must be spread out over a number of periods.

Sometimes the boundary between capital purchases and items that can be allocated to operations in the budget is hazy. However, in accord with legal guidelines for determining what must be capitalized—and consistent with the institution's set of GAAP—the institution generally applies its own guides for determining what should be called a capital purchase. The institution's guide may be expressed as some specific amount of money, some criterion of useful life, or a combination of these. For example, the organization may have decided that any purchased item having a useful life longer than one year and costing more than $200 must be capitalized. Thus a $250 typewriter would be capitalized but a $150 calculator would not, although both will clearly last longer than one year.

The supervisor should learn the institution's guidelines for identifying capital assets. One may either ask for a certain item in the capital budget request or attempt to secure it through the department's expense budget according to where it fits by the organization's definition.

In capital budgeting, requests for purchases often outrun the money available. Requests may come from all directions: from the medical staff, who would like certain equipment to work with; from the public, who would like to see certain services and facilities available; from supervisors and department heads, who would like to have newer and better equipment; and from the government, which may tell the institution that some specific purchase must be made for the sake of conformance with some code, regulation, or requirement.

Development of the capital budget may also involve short-range and long-range capital plans as the institution attempts to determine best what new and replacement equipment will be required for future operations. This process involves looking at all equipment and listing each piece along with its age, original cost, and estimated replacement date. When looking at capital equipment within the specific department, the supervisor should at least list all items according to projected replacement date and then expand this list with proposals for what new equipment may be required in the foreseeable future.

Capital budget requests usually receive close scrutiny, and the request for a substantial capital expenditure usually must be accompanied by the following:

- a realistic assessment of the urgency or priority of the purchase;
- detailed projections of all costs involved in the acquisition;
- a full description of the project and the rationale (justification);
- a statement as to whether the requested item represents an addition, replacement, or improvement;
- the impact, in the case of a revenue-producing department, of the proposed acquisition on revenues.

Most capital budget requests are ordinarily subject to several levels of review and approval. The supervisor may have been assigned a certain dollar limit for capital purchases for the department, but this amount will usually be low when reckoned against the total cost of all desired capital purchases. However, it is just as likely, perhaps even more likely, that the supervisor will personally have no capital budget approval in the department. The supervisor's immediate superior, or perhaps even the administrator or finance director, may retain the authority to approve minimum capital purchases up to a given amount. Many capital expenditures, however, must be authorized by the board of directors. A certain hospital in the eastern United States, a not untypical institution of approximately 200 beds, permits its administrator or finance director to approve capital purchases not exceeding $2,500. Purchases from $2,500 to $10,000 may be approved by the finance committee of the board of directors, and purchases exceeding $10,000 must be approved by the full board.

The Cash Budget

The cash budget is prepared by the accounting department and is usually the last item in the budgeting process. It consists of estimates of the institution's cash needs as compared with projections of cash receipts over the term covered by the budget. The pattern of cash in versus cash out examined in the cash budget is extremely important to the institution because of the need to remain financially solvent in the short run. That is to say, it does little good to appear rich on paper—to have impressive amounts of money owed to the institution—if there is not sufficient cash in the bank to pay today's bills or meet this week's payroll.

The cash budget holds clear implications for everyone concerned with the management of receivables and payables. Should cash be in extremely short supply for a given period, more attention may be turned to the aggressive collection of accounts receivable, or consideration may be given to delaying a few payables until the cash position can better permit payment. A lack of cash can also lead to short-term borrowing, which sometimes results in not inconsiderable difficulties in obtaining credit and leads to still more operating expense because of today's considerable interest rates.

ILLUSTRATION: THE X-RAY DEPARTMENT EXPENSE BUDGET

As an illustration, the expense budget for the x-ray department of a 200-bed hospital will be briefly examined. This budget covers the following:

- personnel expenses (salaries and fringe benefits);
- x-ray film;
- other supplies;
- fixed expenses;
- equipment repairs;
- staff education.

Statistics and Projections

From the projections assembled for the institution as a whole (the statistical budget), the supervisor begins with the following information for the hospital: projected patient days equal 51,500; projected outpatient visits equal 41,000.

In the x-ray department it is known from past experience and through analysis that inpatient tests per day equal 0.2226 and outpatient tests per visit equal 0.3437. Therefore, it can be determined that the department may perform 11,464 inpatient tests and 14,092 outpatient tests, a total of 25,556 tests.

Multiplying time per test by the total number of tests to be performed, it is determined that performance of the department's projected workload will require 33,000 worked hours plus 4,500 nonworked hours or 37,500 hours of personnel time for the budget year.

With projected increases factored in, personnel time for the x-ray department in this illustration is estimated to cost $7 per hour for the budget year. The determination of personnel expense can be far more detailed than this approach suggests. For instance, it is possible to consider each employee in each position, one by one, and apply actual pay rates and add the effects of increases at the precise times they will occur.

The next step involves determining personnel expense for the budget year: $7.00 × 37,500 hours = $262,500.

With regard to elements of cost other than personnel, analysis of film cost and consumption has revealed that an average of 2.40 film units are consumed for each test performed. With a projected price increase being considered, film is expected to cost $2.10 per unit. Therefore:

- 2.40 units per test × 25,556 tests = 61,334 units
- 61,334 units × $2.10 = $128,801.40
- $128,801.40 ÷ 25,556 tests = $5.04 per test.

Concerning other supplies (such as film developer, paper and pencils, labels, or film jackets), variable supply cost analysis shows these costs to amount to $0.671 per test. An eight percent increase in supply costs is expected, so: $0.671 × 1.08 = $0.725 per test for other supplies.

Fixed expenses attributable to the department (perhaps a typewriter maintenance contract, leases on some equipment, and other items that will not vary with activity) have been established through analysis as $18,500 per year.

Further, it has been determined that equipment repairs have historically been costing the department an average of $0.664 per test. It is estimated that a six percent increase in the cost of repairs will be experienced but that there will be no change in repair frequency, so $0.664 times 1.06 equals $0.704 per test repair cost.

Staff education (travel, fees, and other expenses associated with sending employees to educational programs outside of the institution) has been projected at a total of $2,000 for the budget year.

Personnel

One way to handle the personnel portion of the budget is demonstrated in Table 4-1. This method assumes uniform distribution of worked hours at so many per day and assumes distribution of nonworked time on a basis

Table 4-1 Budgeted Personnel Cost Distribution

	33,000 worked hours @ $7	= $231,000
	4,500 nonworked hours @ $7	= 31,500
		$262,500

Month	Days	Time*	Proportion of Total Hours not Worked Nonworked	Projected Cost Worked	Total
January	31	0.0765	$ 1,716	$ 20,719	$ 22,435
February	28	0.0479	1,007	20,010	21,017
March	31	0.0518	1,229	22,492	23,721
April	30	0.0641	1,467	21,414	22,881
May	31	0.0707	1,603	21,068	22,671
June	30	0.0935	2,209	21,412	23,621
July	31	0.1129	2,358	18,528	20,886
August	31	0.1295	2,735	18,387	21,122
September	30	0.1116	2,313	18,415	20,728
October	31	0.0602	1,302	20,319	21,621
November	30	0.0842	1,739	18,910	20,649
December	31	0.0971	2,053	19,095	21,148
	365	1.0000	$ 21,731	$ 240,769	$262,500

*Determined from historical information modified by expected vacation time.

suggested by past practice and knowledge of some future events (such as personnel scheduling). One could conceivably do a more accurate job of spreading the personnel budget if one had knowledge of a pattern of fluctuation in department activity such as that occurring in institutions in which the workload is subject to seasonal fluctuations.

Film, Other Supplies, and Equipment Repairs

The month-by-month projection of these three items of expense that are reasonably believed to vary with workload is listed in Table 4-2. Thus a month with 30 days will absorb a slightly smaller portion of such expense than will a month with 31 days.

Fixed Expense

The $18,500 fixed expense for the year is spread evenly by simply assigning one-twelfth of that total to each month of the budget year.

Staff Education

The $2,000 for staff education is spread evenly across the budget year. Granted this amount is not likely to be consumed in the same pattern in which

Table 4-2 Film, Other Supplies, and Equipment Repairs

Month	Total Tests	Film Cost @ $5.04/Test	Other Supplies @ $0.725/Test	Repairs @ $0.704/Test
January	2,185	$ 11,012	$ 1,584	$ 1,538
February	2,048	10,322	1,485	1,442
March	2,310	11,642	1,675	1,626
April	2,228	11,229	1,615	1,569
May	2,206	11,118	1,599	1,553
June	2,300	11,592	1,668	1,619
July	2,034	10,251	1,475	1,432
August	2,057	10,367	1,491	1,448
September	2,017	10,166	1,462	1,420
October	2,104	10,604	1,525	1,481
November	2,009	10,125	1,457	1,414
December	2,058	10,372	1,492	1,449
	25,556	$ 128,800	$ 18,528	$ 17,991

it is budgeted, but as long as the education money is spent throughout the year with that budget limit in mind, the results will be satisfactory. This amount could be budgeted more accurately if one had information about expected patterns of attendance at programs; for example, a department may always send two people to the same annual conference in the same month each year. The results, however, should prove satisfactory as long as the year's expenditures remain within the total. Note also that this amount of money is completely manageable by the supervisor since it is usually at the supervisor's discretion that employees are permitted to attend outside programs.

The X-Ray Department Expense Budget

Exhibit 4-1 represents the expense budget for the x-ray department for the year. One need not be reminded that a departmental budget is far from precise. Close examination of this illustration will reveal some gaps. For example, predicting equipment repairs as a function of number of tests is a questionable practice because there is little solid evidence to use. Repair cost might just as well have been spread evenly over the months. Note, however, that manageable items of cost, such as staff education, are better highlighted by the budget and placed before the supervisor where they can be controlled in relation to the way other expenses are perceived.

Consider also those expenses that are partly manageable, such as personnel. There are many management actions that can be taken when actual cost and activity begin to move one way or another. One may wish to permit or even encourage the heaviest use of vacation time during periods when workload falls off. Also, by highlighting all elements of cost in the depart-

Exhibit 4-1 X-Ray Department Expense Budget

	Jan.	Feb.	March	April	May	June	July	Aug.	Sept.	Oct.	Nov.	Dec.	Totals
Salaries and Wages	22,435	21,017	23,721	22,881	22,671	23,621	20,886	21,122	20,728	21,621	20,649	21,148	262,500
Film	11,102	10,322	11,642	11,229	11,118	11,592	10,251	10,367	10,166	10,604	10,125	10,372	128,800
Other Supplies	1,584	1,485	1,675	1,615	1,599	1,668	1,475	1,491	1,462	1,525	1,457	1,492	18,528
Repairs	1,538	1,442	1,626	1,569	1,553	1,619	1,432	1,448	1,420	1,481	1,414	1,449	17,991
Fixed Expense	1,542	1,542	1,542	1,542	1,542	1,542	1,542	1,542	1,542	1,542	1,542	1,542	18,504
Staff Education	167	167	167	167	167	167	167	167	167	167	167	167	2,004
Total	38,278	35,975	40,373	39,003	38,650	40,209	35,753	36,137	35,485	36,940	35,354	36,170	448,327

ment, the budget supplies the basis for ongoing awareness of supply expenses and other variable costs. Should the supervisor see the cost of supplies suddenly exceeding the projected amount, he or she will be alert to the need for investigation and possible action. Without a budget, certain costs could run excessively high for months without the supervisor's awareness of the situation.

A budget is a plan. As such it attempts to look into a time in the future, and it is necessarily based on estimates and projections. It is not ever to be regarded as a preordained, concrete picture of future events. Rarely will the budget be precisely as it should have been budgeted, and rarely will the results be exactly as predicted. In this respect the budget is much like any other management tool: it cannot do the management job, but probably a better management job can result with it than without it.

THE BUDGETING PROCESS

Responsibilities

The responsibility for preparing the budget rests in part with each of several individuals and groups:

The *board of directors* is ultimately responsible for everything in the budget and thus retains the authority for its final approval. Although the board is not likely to become involved in the details of budget preparation, this body will probably rule on proposed capital expenditures item by item and review and approve the principal parts of the budget. The board role in the approval of the budget is consistent wth the directors' legal responsibilities as trustees of the resources of the organization.

The *administrator* must assure that the budget being submitted to the board is consistent with the goals of the organization and is realistic and workable in the light of current knowledge of expected revenues and expenses.

The *finance director* has an active role in preparing the cash and revenue budgets and assembling all pieces of the operating budget into a total budget for the institution. Like the administrator, the finance director must assure that budgeting guidelines are followed and that the resulting plan appears to be workable and realistic for what is known about the coming budget year.

All *supervisors* and *department heads*, at least under a participative budgeting approach, are responsible for assembling the expense and capital budgets for their own departments. In accounting or budgeting terms, the smallest organizational unit for which a budget is prepared is usually identified as a "cost center." A cost center, an organizational unit for which costs are identified and collected, is usually provided with expense and capital budgets prepared by the supervisor. In the case of middle- or upper-level managers who may have charge of several cost centers, the task also includes assembling individual cost center budgets into a budget for their total areas of responsiblity.

A *budget committee* may be established each year to facilitate the preparation of the budget. This committee will usually consist of the administrator, the finance director, the director of nursing service and other department heads, and perhaps a member of the finance committee of the board of directors. It is the role of the budget committee to establish and distribute the guidelines for budget preparation, to decide how particular problems should be solved and certan issues dealt with as they occur, and to keep all stages of budget preparation actively moving toward completion.

The Budget Coordination Meeting

The budget coordination meeting is generally seen as a kickoff for the year's activity in putting together the budget. If the target for presentation to the boad should be sometime in October, the budget coordination meeting may take place in June or July. Convened and conducted by members of the budget committee, the coordination meeting should include all managers who have an active role in budget preparation. At this meeting the most recent volume factors are introduced, policies affecting budgeting are reviewed and any changes are noted, planned organizational changes likely to affect budgeting factors are viewed and clarified, and trends of likely future activity are discussed. In short, any known or suspected factor that may have a bearing on the budget's preparation is reviewed.

Many institutions use a budget manual, a book of informational and instructional documents assembled under the guidance of the budget committee for the current year's budget preparation activity. Given to the person who must prepare and present a budget for one or more cost centers, this manual contains all information, instructions, and forms necessary for budget preparation.

The budget manual describes the full scope and purpose of the budgeting program; outlines all procedures for preparation, review, and revision of budgets; and defines the duties, authority, and responsiblity of all persons involved in the process.

The Budget Calendar

The preparation of the budget for a sizeable health care institution is an exercise in timing. Budgets for dozens of individual cost centers must be put together, and these must be assembled into budgets for the larger organizational units and eventually into a budget for the total institution. If two or three pieces of the buildup are missing, the total budget is delayed. Also, the cash budget cannot be properly prepared until the operating and capital budgets are complete.

The budget calendar displays deadline dates for all steps in the budget preparation process. The calendar will let a supervisor know when the department's draft budget must be submitted, when it is likely to be returned following initial review, when the revision must be submitted, and how much time must be allowed for the approval process.

Much of the trauma that can be encountered in the annual budgeting exercise is a result of matters of timing. We often tend to get things done at the deadline or perhaps even a little late, and our planning rarely anticipates all contingencies. As a result, it is often necessary to go through the whole process again, perhaps several times, on the way to a realistic, workable budget for the entire institution. Dozens of supervisors can enter the budgeting process with the best of intentions, yet the results may be unsatisfactory the first time around because the key persons assembling the final budget do not know exactly where the totals are going to fall until all the pieces are put together for the first time. The process then enters into a period of back-and-forth activity as efforts are made to shift resources in more appropriate directions to make it possible to come up with a realistic budget.

Review and Coordination

When all of the individual departments' draft budgets are submitted, the accounting department will prepare the total budget for approval of the estimates. As already suggested, the budget may go through several drafts before the budget committee believes it has a document appropriate for submission to the board of directors.

Adoption

A summary of the total budget will be presented to the board of directors for discussion and approval. This summary generally includes:

- a narrative description of the budget, some of its key elements, and the reasons behind its preparation;
- a condensed income statement for the budget year;
- a summary of capital expenditure requests;
- a cash analysis covering the budget period;
- the key factors in forecasting;
- estimates of the impact of this budget on the institution's services and finances.

The board of directors will either approve or reject the budget in whole or in part as the trustees see fit. Necessary elements of the process are repeated until the board approves a budget for the coming year. Most health care institutions that operate on a calendar fiscal year (January 1–December 31) will attempt to secure approval of the coming year's budget at either the November or December meeting of the board of directors. Occasionally problems encountered in coming up with a workable budget make approval impossible in the desired time, and the institution may enter the new year working against a tentative or provisional budget that may ultimately meet with full board approval one, two, or three months into the year.

"FINISHED" IS JUST BEGUN

A budget should be a live, working plan. For it to serve in this capacity, timely and accurate reporting of operating results is required.

Reporting the results of operations is generally a responsibility of the accounting department. Timeliness is essential: the more recent the feedback received on results, the more valuable the budget is in highlighting the need for management action. The information received each month—a comparison of operating results for the period with the budget projections for the period—allows the supervisor to make adjustments for those aspects of operations that are wholly or partly under direct supervisory control.

Reporting is often done in a way that highlights exceptions, that is, the reporting system, built on recognition of the likely presence of natural variations between operating results and budget projections, will specifically flag the items that appear to be out of line beyond normal variation.

A Sample Budget Report

Exhibit 4-2 is a sample budget report, identified as an *operating expenses schedule*, taken from the personnel department of a hospital in the 400- to 500-bed range. In two sections it deals separately with personnel expenses (technician and specialist labor, and clerical and administrative labor) and non-labor expenses (all costs of running the personnel department other than salaries and wages). (Absent from consideration are employee benefit costs, which are separately budgeted in a benefits cost center.)

From left to right the columns on the schedule represent: identifying numbers of the individual accounts; the department using the accounts; the names of the accounts; actual expenditures charged to each account for the month under consideration; the amounts budgeted for the month; the variances for the month (the differences between actual and budgeted) in both absolute dollars and percentage of budget; and, for the year to date, the actual expenditures, the budgeted amounts, and the variances for each account.

In the *actual* columns the occasional minus sign after a dollar amount indicates a credit to an account. In Exhibit 4-2 the negative amount for account 901, Dues and Subscriptions, reflects a refund received on cancellation of a prepaid subscription service.

The minus signs in the *variance* columns have a different meaning. A minus sign after a variance dollar amount indicates a favorable variance, a condition of being under budget by that amount. Thus a minus sign after a variance percentage also indicates a favorable variance; the account stands at that percent under budget.

Caution is in order regarding the use of minus signs in budget reports. Their use is not always consistent from organization to organization. But minus signs carry a generally negative connotation for many people, a connotation that is often the reverse of their meaning in a budget report. In Exhibit 4-2, and indeed in many organizations' budget reports, the minus sign attached to a variance is good in that it means *under*, a condition of being under the budgeted amount

Exhibit 4-2 Operating Expenses Schedule
Period Ending 03/31/84

			----------THIS MONTH----------			--------- YEAR TO DATE ---------			
Department-937		Actual	Budget	Variance	Pct	Actual	Budget	Variance	Pct
502 Personnel Dept	Technician & Spe	10,812.03	10,758.09	53.94	1	31,543.27	31,663.16	119.89	0
506 Personnel Dept	Clerical & Admin	8,814.42	8,715.30	99.12	1	25,915.60	25,650.86	264.70	1
		19,626.45	19,473.39	153.06	1	57,458.87	57,314.02	144.85	0
545 Personnel Dept	Prof Serv Purch	0.00	83.30	83.30-	100-	0.00	249.90	249.90	100-
571 Personnel Dept	Emp Ed & Train	390.00	499.80	109.80-	22-	1,233.61	1,499.40	265.79-	18-
711 Personnel Dept	Misc Food Items	98.47	0.00	98.47	0	98.47	0.00	98.47	0
759 Personnel Dept	Books & Film	58.50	63.53	5.03-	8-	78.45	186.43	107.98-	58-
763 Personnel Dept	Office Supplies	167.88	152.46	15.42	10	258.52	447.48	161.96-	36-
769 Personnel Dept	Misc General Sup	152.39	0.00	152.39	0	221.00	0.00	221.00	0
787 Personnel Dept	Inv Chg-Inst,Med	0.00	0.00	0.00	0	4.26	0.00	4.26	0
789 Personnel Dept	Inv Chg-Dietary	2.03	25.41	23.38-	92-	15.61-	74.58	58.97-	79-
794 Personnel Dept	Inv Chg-Forms, P	129.91	127.05	2.86	2	196.52	372.90	176.38-	47-
796 Personnel Dept	Inv Chg-Office S	65.68	50.82	14.86	29	173.68	149.16	24.52	16
797 Personnel Dept	Inv Chg-Paper Go	2.43	2.12	0.31	15	6.57	6.20	0.37	6
798 Personnel Dept	Inv Chg-Miscell a	47.99	4.24	43.75	32	97.38	12.41	84.97	685
805 Personnel Dept	Prevent Mtc Cont	0.00	125.70	125.70-	100-	233.75	363.75	130.00-	36-
809 Personnel Dept	Misc Repair	0.00	20.95	20.95-	100-	0.00	60.60	60.60-	100-
867 Personnel Dept	Photocopy Charge	64.30	100.56	36.26-	36-	251.35	291.00	39.65-	14-
901 Personnel Dept	Dues & Subscript	170.00-	263.97	433.97-	164-	597.25	763.85	166.60-	22-
907 Personnel Dept	Postage	5.87	8.47	2.60-	31-	15.62	24.86	9.24-	37-
913 Personnel Dept	Public Relations	2.00	49.98	47.98-	96-	5.75	149.94	144.19-	96-
931 Personnel Dept	Misc Other Expen	17.62-	0.00	17.62-	0	6.00-	0.00	6.00-	0
		999.83	1,578.36	578.53-	37-	3,508.79	4,652.46	1,143.67-	25-
		20,626.28	21,051.75	425.47-	2-	60,967.66	61,966.48	998.82-	2-

In analyzing a budget report it is best to begin with the obvious. In the case of Exhibit 4-2 the obvious consists of those accounts for which there are charges but no budget.

It often happens that charges appear against a zero budget, that is, an account for which the department has budgeted no expenditures. This occurs because persons in the department make errors filling out requisitions and other forms, and because persons filling out forms may not provide sufficient detail and others are left to place the charges in specific accounts. In the exhibit, the charge to account 711, Miscellaneous Food Items, was found to be an error; another department should have been charged.

The supervisor should assure that all the department's employees who trigger expenditures and charges supply full charging information. This full information usually includes both department number and specific account number. In the exhibit, the $152.39 incorrectly charged to account 769 came from paperwork that indicated only department 937 in the "Charge to" space; someone in the accounting department made a guess as to the account number. The accounting manager might concede that his clerk could have called the personnel department to learn the correct account number. He could also claim some justification, however, that he would have to increase the size of his staff significantly to be able to call for every missing account number. The difficulty could have been avoided in the first place if the initiating personnel department employee had been required to enter the number 937-763 under "Charge to."

Occasionally, charges to accounts for which there is no budget may be legitimate. If the account in question appears to be the most logical place for a particular charge but there is no budget, this should serve as a flag to consider that account as a legitimate line item for the coming budget year (if it appears that such charges may occur again).

The supervisor is often provided with guidelines for analyzing the budget report and answering for variances. Such guidelines are usually expressed as a variance threshold beyond which answers are expected. For example, the guidelines for the manager of the personnel department of Exhibit 4-2 are:

- For personnel costs, explanation or justification must be provided for variances beyond (+) or (−) two percent *or* (+) or (−) $1,000 for total departmental personnel cost for the month.
- For nonpersonnel expense, explanation or justification must be provided for variances beyond (+) or (−) ten percent *or* (+) or (−) $50 for any specific account for the month.

It is almost as important to answer to variances under budget as to variances over budget. A condition of under budget for a period does not necessarily mean that money is being saved or that a favorable condition is emerging. It can often indicate that expenditures are occurring in a pattern inconsistent with the budget allocation, and it can sometimes indicate that certain necessary or desirable expenditures have been overlooked.

Under a thorough financial control system the supervisor is usually expected to answer to his or her immediate superior for budget variances. Exhibit 4-3 is a sample budget variance report for the personnel department of Exhibit 4-2. Exhibit 4-3 shows the personnel manager's response to the first several items of concern on Exhibit 4-2—those first items that fall beyond the (+) or (−) ten percent or (+) or (−) $50 threshold for the month.

In addition to being provided with a monthly report of expenditures versus budget, the supervisor usually receives detailed backup as to the individual

Exhibit 4-3 Budget Variance Report
Month of March 1984

Dept. Name	Dept. No.	Manager	Responsible V.P.
Personnel	937	J.W. Johnson	R.B. Perry

Sub Acct. No.	Variance	Reason	Action to Be Taken & Anticipated Outcome
545	100% under	Account for professional service purchased—temporary help. No expenses yet this year.	Anticipate no use of account until vacation coverage required during July.
571	22% under	Behind schedule on sending staff to conferences.	Will reach zero variance by end of June with charges for annual personnel seminar.
763	10% over (but should be 110% over)	First-quarter special supply order billed in March. Next month's expense will be minimal. WIth error in 769 corrected, should show 110% over for month & −2% YTD.	2% under budget year to date. Anticipate finishing year 15% under budget.
789	92% under	Charges occur unevenly throughout the year—heaviest activity to come (refreshments for retirement planning sessions in fall).	No action necessary.
796	29% over	Unusually high use rate for pads, pens, etc.	Altering procedures to call for dept. secretary to issue (as well as order) supplies. Should see change in a month if any of usage is "leakage."

Note: Comments should note if one-time variance, constant variance, or potential escalating variance and action to be taken.

YTD = year to date.

charges made to each account. This backup aids the supervisor in assessing the validity of most charges.

In working with budget reports the supervisor should make a habit of questioning all details that are not completely understood. Learning month by month where all of the department's budget dollars are going will eventually enable the supervisor to alter at least partially patterns of expenditure to improve unfavorable trends that appear to be developing.

CONTROL: AWARENESS PLUS ACTION

Preparing a budget and working with it throughout the year heightens the supervisor's awareness of how the department's resources, for which the supervisor is responsible, are used in fulfilling the department's responsibilities. Reports of actual results versus budget projections provide all-important information on which to base corrective action when needed. For instance, when productivity problems occur and the relationship between worked hours and the volume of work begins to change unfavorably, the supervisor can take positive steps that might include effective use of overtime, the application of call time, scheduling of vacations and other time off, and routine scheduling of personnel for day-to-day coverage.

Viewing the budget and feedback on actual operations from the perspective of a complete organizational unit—whether a small department or an entire institution—consider what is obtained from the process: at any time you know *where you are* relative to *where you thought you might be*, and you also know where to look for improvement.

Part III

Productivity: Getting More from the Same or the Same from Less

Chapter 5

The What and Why of Productivity

Productivity is the first test of management's competence.

Peter F. Drucker

Chapter Objectives

- Offer a working definition of productivity and establish productivity improvement as more than simple "cost cutting."
- Review health care productivity relative to productivity within the general economy.
- Establish the relationship between productivity improvement and health care cost inflation.
- Develop an understanding of the individual supervisor's responsibility for continuing improvement of productivity.

PRODUCTIVITY DEFINED

Productivity may be described as the level of output obtained from the application of a given amount of input, that is, productivity is the relationship, expressed as either a percentage or a ratio, between output and input. It is a measure of the efficiency with which goods and services are produced. Stated in its most elementary form: resources are fed into a system or process, something (usually a conversion of form or substance) takes place within that system or process, and some form of product or services comes out. This elementary chain of events is depicted in Figure 5-1.

Usually expressed as a percentage, the relationship between output and input, and thus the basic productivity relationship, is simply:

$$\frac{\text{Output}}{\text{Input}} \times 100 = \text{percent efficiency, or productivity.}$$

Productivity improvement is often thought of as "cost cutting," in effect, maintaining output while trimming input and thus forcing the resulting percentage to grow. It can indeed be true that productivity grows when output is held constant and input is reduced, but productivity also increases when:

- Output is increased while input is held constant.
- Output and input both increase, but output increases at a faster rate than input.

Figure 5-1 From Resources to Product or Service

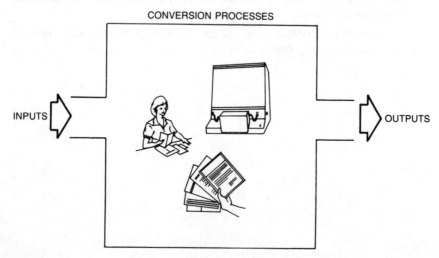

- Output and input both decrease, but output decreases at a slower rate than input.

Our thinking concerning the basic productivity relationship should not be limited to assumed constant forms of input and output. Productivity can be altered by changing forms of output—perhaps abandoning some products or services for the sake of offering others—and by changing forms of input— perhaps by replacing costly human labor with automation or by changing the mix of skills in the work force. The basic productivity relationship is simple, but the combinations of ways in which this relationship may be altered in a complex, modern health care organization are almost infinite.

THE IMPORTANCE OF PRODUCTIVITY

During the 1950s and 1960s productivity improvement in the American economy was healthy and consistent. During that 20-year period productivity in the farm sector of the economy grew at an average rate of 5.8 percent per year. In trade and manufacturing average productivity growth was 2.9 percent per year. In some unmeasured areas of the economy, including health care, productivity growth was estimated at slightly less than 2.9 percent but generally more than 2.0 percent. For several decades total productivity in the American economy grew at an average rate of 3.2 percent per year.[1]

However, about 1970 the overall rate of growth of American productivity decreased to approximately 1.0 percent per year. Although more than once showing signs of partially recovering in an up-and-down pattern, in general American productivity declined through the 1970s and growth rates lagged behind those of most other industrialized nations. In the latter half of 1979 total productivity actually experienced a negative growth rate (that is, not only did productivity fail to rise during that period, it actually fell below the previous period's level).[2] Through the 1970s periodic modest surges in productivity were complicated by rising wages and prices and by growing unemployment, and, as always, lagging productivity both contributed to and resulted from increases in wages, prices, and unemployment.

Through the 1970s health care costs increased considerably faster than overall inflation, yet health care productivity did not grow at as fast a rate as productivity grew in most other segments of the economy.[3]

A known way of restraining inflation is to increase productivity. Since this is so, the reverse is generally held to be true, that rising rates of inflation exert some forces that have the effect of restricting productivity growth. The relationship between productivity and inflation has been well demonstrated in health care; health care has for years had the highest inflation rate and one of the lowest productivity growth rates in the American economy.

PRODUCTIVITY AND INFLATION

As long as the increases that economic entities, including people, receive for the products and services they supply are not fully matched by increases in what they produce, inflationary pressures are being created. When a single inflationary pressure is created, for example, that caused by a collective bargaining organization that secures a pay increase for its members without requiring increased output, or that caused when the price of a product is increased without a corresponding increase in buyers' ability to pay for the product, the difference must be made up by other units of the economy. Figure 5-2 shows that when input grows at a faster rate than output, the result is lower productivity, and the resulting pressures tend to hold output down and to artificially increase input.

Every economic entity, whether individual, labor union, corporation, or government, has its own "productivity equation." All such entities buy the outputs of others as their inputs and sell their outputs to be used as others' inputs. A demand for an increase in input, although it may be fully understandable but nevertheless unjustified by appropriate increases in output, is in effect the demanding economic entity saying: "I know what *I* need, but I cannot concern myself with what happens in *your* input-output equation as a result."

Figure 5-2 The Inflationary Spiral of Lagging Productivity Growth

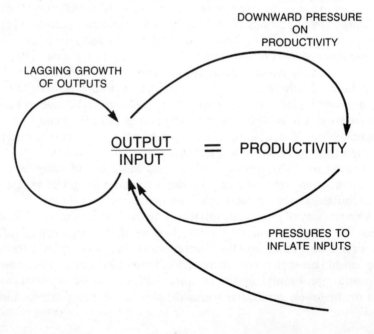

Individual economic entities, however, do not stand alone. Increases in output that are not justified—are not "bought"—by increases in productivity ultimately have an effect on the input-output equation of every economic entity.

THE SUPERVISOR'S RELATIONSHIP TO PRODUCTIVITY

Three dimensions of productivity are highly relevant to the health care institution. These are the dimensions of institutional, technological, and personnel productivity.

Institutional Productivity

Institutional productivity is determined by any number of the actions of the organization as a health care provider. Included are the efficiency of management, the utilization of services, the development of alternatives to hospitalization, wellness programs and other treatment-avoidance efforts, and participation in affiliations and multi-institutional arrangements. In short, anything the institution can do to alter its total input or output can have an impact on institutional productivity.

Technological Productivity

Technological productivity is determined by the interrelationships of the patterns of development, introduction, and utilization of new medical practices, equipment, and drugs. One technological innovation may be more or less productive than another in the outputs achieved relative to the inputs it requires. Technological productivity of course often affects institutional productivity; an institution adopting a new practice takes into its total productivity relationship the relative productivity of that practice.

Personnel Productivity

Personnel productivity is determined by the application of personnel time, skill, and effort to delivering the services of the institution.

These three major dimensions of health care institution productivity are inseparably interrelated; one cannot exist without the others, and it is not possible to alter one without affecting the others in some way. To bring these dimensions more into common focus: The organization decides what kind of provider it is and what services it will offer (the institutional dimension); decisions are made as to how—in a medical and technical sense—these services will be delivered (the technological dimension); and decisions are made as to who—people of what skills, how many of them, and how best to utilize their time and abilities—will deliver the services (the personnel dimension).

It is frequently said that management is "getting things done through people." In accomplishing this aim, the supervisor is there to assure that proper methods are followed and to provide guidance to the employees so they can put forth their best efforts and produce the desired quality in the most efficient manner. The individual supervisor can have great impact on productivity; indeed, it is a large part of the supervisor's role to enhance productivity through upward pressure on output and downward pressure on input, and always to try to accomplish the best possible results with the minimum essential resources. In addition to managing the efforts of the employees, the supervisor should seek to exercise a voice in determining the directions taken by the institution and in deciding on the application of new technology.

Productivity Incentives

Overall, long-run increases in productivity within health care will require incentives for both providers and consumers. Providers (organizations and individuals alike) need incentives to provide quality health care at competitive prices. Consumers need incentives to become more interested in self-care and disease prevention, to seek to know more about their health care, and to question available alternatives. After years of attempting to deal with rising health care costs through increased productivity and other means, it would appear that the most effective incentives, particularly as applied to providers of health care, are financial.

A 1980 report by the National Council on Health Planning and Development concluded in part that:

> changes in existing reimbursement methodologies should be pursued for both professionals and institutions. In the case of professionals, "usual, customary and reasonable" (UCR) reimbursement or "fee schedule" reimbursement should be revised to include incentives for productivity. In the case of institutions, retrospective "cost-based" and "charge-based" reimbursement should be revised to include incentives for productivity.[4]

It is precisely in the direction suggested in the National Council report that the new Medicare reimbursement system is taking institutional providers of health care, and similar efforts are being undertaken to regulate the income of individual professionals as well. The most pressing reason why persons in health care should be interested in productivity improvement is thus the cost containment pressure created by nationwide introduction of prospective pricing.[5]

The 1984 implementation of the Medicare reimbursement system places many hospitals under a form of prospective payment for the first time. In states that until 1984 had remained essentially unregulated, a number of hospitals will experience financial pressure stemming from payment for a large part of their patient population. Medicare accounts for about 36 percent of all hospital operating revenue, and Medicare reimbursement rates will now be determined completely independently of individual hospital costs.[6]

Simply stated, when cost mattered less, improvement of productivity was not seen as a very pressing need. But with cost now assuming a position of importance nearly equal to quality of care, the enhancement of productivity assumes high priority. Since there will likely be no reversal in the trend toward total control of medical costs, the new emphasis on productivity improvement is essentially permanent.

Focus of Responsibility

The individual supervisor should always take an interest in the direction pursued by the organization as a whole and should provide input into planning processes whenever possible. However, the supervisor ultimately has little control over the determination of services to be offered, populations to be served, and organizational goals to pursue. Likewise, the individual supervisor may have nominal input but little control regarding the technology that is adopted to aid in delivering service. The lone first-line supervisor has only a small amount of control over institutional productivity and technological productivity; these remain the responsibility of administration and the board of directors.

However, the individual supervisor, in guiding and working with the employees in the work group, can exercise maximum control of personnel productivity. A great deal of productivity improvement has to occur at the points where human and material resources are actually applied in the rendering of hands-on patient care. Although administration and the board of directors essentially supply the framework within which all others can be most productive, it is the individual supervisor's or manager's primary responsiblity to make the institution's care-delivery processes as productive as possible.

NOTES

1. U.S. Bureau of the Census, *Statistical Abstract* (Washington, D.C.: GPO, 1970–1980).
2. National Council on Health Planning and Development, *Productivity and Health*, DHHS Publication no. (HRA)80–14022, p. 3.
3. Ibid.
4. Ibid., p. 17.
5. Glenn Richards, "Working Smarter: Productivity Takes On New Importance under Prospective Pricing," *Hospitals*, October 1, 1983, p. 92.

Chapter 6

Measuring and Monitoring Productivity

We are too much inclined to measure progress by the billions spent rather than by the work completed.

Anonymous

Chapter Objectives

- Introduce the key consideration in measuring productivity, that of valuing output and input in comparable terms.
- Review the advantages and disadvantages of the various methods of establishing productivity standards.
- Outline and illustrate a representative procedure for establishing a departmental productivity standard.
- Establish the supervisor's role in measuring and monitoring departmental productivity.

MEASURING PRODUCTIVITY

Productivity, expressed as the ratio of output to input, is simple in concept and readily understood. Productivity measurement, however, is quite another matter; the application of the concept in a manner that produces reliable and credible numbers is frequently difficult and involved.

Productivity measurement remains as simple as understanding the concept of productivity only in those few instances in which output and input take precisely the same form. Consider the simple example of electrical power transmission. The operator of an electrical power transmission line can accurately determine the efficiency or productivity of that line by metering the electricity flowing from the end of the line and comparing this output with the metered amount of electricity flowing into the line. A certain amount of electricity goes into the line, a certain amount of electricity flows from the line, and the drop in output from input is measurable and can be associated with known forms of transmission loss. Thus the efficiency or productivity of the line can be determined.

However, beyond simple physical examples such as that of the electrical power transmission line, outputs and inputs are usually vastly different from each other. Beyond the realm of the physical and in the domain of the economic, outputs and inputs are virtually guaranteed to differ because economic activities—that is, the production of goods and services—essentially involve the conversion of certain resources into other desired forms. Thus the manufacturer converts skills and labor and metals and other raw material into manufactured products; the attorney-at-law converts knowledge and skill into legal services; the cook transforms labor and skill and raw food into meals; and the health care provider converts knowledge and skill and various supplies into medical services.

The system of the institutional health care provider operates on two basic inputs—the patient who is in need of service, and the money that pays for the knowledge and skill and supplies that are needed to serve that patient. This system produces but a single output, the patient who leaves the system in a state different from that experienced on entering.

Since output and input are usually so different from each other, any attempt at direct comparison is bound to be as pointless as comparing apples with oranges. For appropriate comparison of output with input, and thus for the measurement of productivity, it is necessary to find a way to value output and input in common terms. In productivity measurement the common term ordinarily used for valuing both input and output is *time*.

Lest this discussion be perceived as ignoring the most important single characteristic of the delivery of health care, a few words are in order about quality of care versus productivity. We must always consider the maintenance or improvement of the quality of care as the overriding constraint on the health care delivery system. However, the concept of productivity is not inconsistent with quality. There are many prevailing misconceptions concerning the relationship between quality and quantity of output; there is a strong tendency for many people to believe that *any* change in practice that increases quantity must necessarily diminish quality. The age-old admonition that haste makes waste does indeed apply at times, but it generally applies only after a point that many human activities have not yet reached.

Consider the simple graphic representation of Figure 6-1. This generalized curve suggests that there is an ideal point (A) at which quality and quantity are in balance; optimum quality exists in a relationship with a certain level of output. Beyond this point on the output scale (at point B, for example) haste does indeed make waste. The quality-versus-quantity trap lies in the tendency to believe that a given activity is already being conducted at the optimum quality point (A). In actuality, however, the majority of work activities take place along the rising curve at some point (C, for example) below the optimum combination of quality and output. In other words, there

Figure 6-1 Quality versus Output

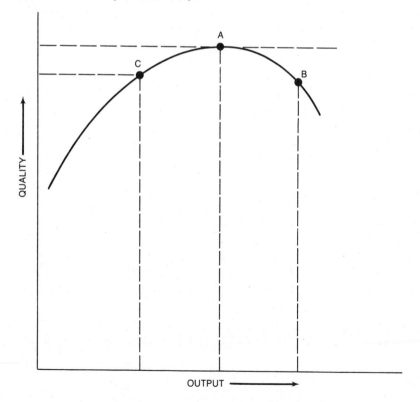

remains in most activities room for productivity improvement that can be achieved while maintaining or improving quality.

To accept intuitively the premise of Figure 6-1, the supervisor need consider only the relationship between the department's individual workers and the quality they produce. Is the best quality work produced by those employees who are slowest? Usually not. Ordinarily it is the faster workers, those who keep up with the requirements of the job and produce sufficient quantities of work, who turn out work of consistently acceptable quality.

The primary input into any business operation is money, the ultimate resource used for the acquisition of all the other resources that go into the production of goods and services. The resources of production can be further subdivided into two general kinds: human labor and all physical resources (such as buildings, equipment, raw materials, supplies).

To measure productivity effectively it is necessary to measure the utilization of both human and physical resources. Since physical resources are tangible items to which specific price tags can be attached, and, further, since their use is generally controlled by human effort, their worth and contribution are measurable fairly easily. Human labor, however, is another matter. Labor is generally the controlling input in the production of most goods and services, and certainly is so in the production of health care services; to measure productivity effectively in health care, it is necessary to measure objectively the controlling input of human labor and to value output in the same terms.

Human labor can be measured by the application of stopwatch time study, the use of predetermined motion times, work sampling and other statistically based techniques, or the use of productivity targets, guidelines, or benchmarks. These processes and their advantages and disadvantages are described as follows:

1) *Stopwatch time study.* This process develops productivity standards through direct observation and repeated timing of work activities by persons trained in techniques of analyzing jobs and timing elements of work. The advantages of this approach are:

- Work standards resulting from stopwatch time study are among the most accurate that can be developed.
- Since time study must be accomplished at the job site, the analyst becomes completely involved in the intimate details of the work.
- The detailed information provided by stopwatch time study usually makes it possible to analyze specific tasks in minute detail when necessary.

The disadvantages of this approach are:

- It is expensive and time consuming to set stopwatch time standards for all of the tasks in a complex operation.
- The technique is of limited applicability to tasks that are nonrepetitive in nature.
- Since it requires direct observation of people at work and involves the obvious recording of their activities, stopwatch time study frequently creates problems in employee relations.

2) *Predetermined motion times.* Standard building blocks of time associated with basic human motions used in the performance of work are applied. A number of specific systems are available, the best known of which is probably Methods-Time Measurement (MTM). Application requires the work analyst to observe an activity in detail but without timing the work. Times are applied from a catalog of basic motion times after a task has been thoroughly analyzed. Predetermined time approaches also include the use of semicustomized time standards developed using generalized systems like MTM in conjunction with stopwatch time study and specialized knowledge of particular tasks to create time standards that apply only to specific kinds of tasks found in specific activities or industries. Some examples of such systems include the College of American Pathologists (CAP) laboratory standards and the various departmental methodologies making up the Resource Monitoring System (RMS) of the Hospital Association of New York State. The major advantages of predetermined motion time systems are:

- They produce reasonably accurate standards, with the accuracy of the generalized systems (such as MTM) and even some of the specialized systems (such as RMS) closely approaching the accuracy of stopwatch time study.
- Since on-the-spot observation is required, time standards can be tailored to a specific working situation.
- In some applications they can provide accurate standards at considerably less cost than stopwatch time study (this applies largely to the specialized approaches designed for application within specific hospital departments).
- The processes are fully as applicable to nonrepetitive work as they are to repetitive work.
- Although direct observation of employees is necessary, it is usually more acceptable than stopwatch time study because no timing is involved.

The disadvantages of predetermined motion times include:

- Application of the generalized approaches (again, such as MTM) can be as costly and time consuming as stopwatch time study.
- The amount of time and effort and thus the amount of cost that must be put into developing a standard for a nonrepetitive, occasional task may outweigh the value of productivity improvements to be realized from that task.
- Since times are applied from fixed values independently of work observation, standards set by predetermined motion times are generally vulnerable to perceptions suggesting that many of the subtleties involved in performing work are absent from consideration.

3) *Work sampling*. This is a process by which a statistically sound number of observations are made at random frequencies to determine the percentage of time that an individual (and often a group) spends on each of a number of given activities. The advantages of work sampling include:

- It is generally a less expensive technique than those previously discussed.
- It is applicable to a broad range of human activity.
- It can be competently applied by a work analyst upon considerably less training than is required by either stopwatch time study or predetermined motion times.
- For many highly repetitive and moderately repetitive activities it is the most economical work measurement technique so far discussed.
- It is highly applicable to the study of indirect labor or support-type activities.

The disadvantages of work sampling are:

- It is impractical and disproportionately costly to use in setting standards for occasional, nonrepetitive tasks, since the number of observations required to assure standards of reasonable statistical validity cannot be secured within reasonable time or with reasonable effort.
- Standards developed through work sampling are generally less accurate than standards developed by stopwatch time study or by using predetermined motion times.
- Since the process does not involve prolonged work observation at any particular time but rather relies on spot observations, rarely is the analyst able to develop a fully detailed picture of how all of the elements of

a task connect. This limits the analyst's ability to recognize potential improvements in methods.

4) *Guidelines, targets, or benchmarks.* Hardly worthy of being dignified by the label of standards but nevertheless applied as standards of sorts in many institutions, productivity guidelines, targets, or benchmarks are used by many organizations. Some of these come from published statistical reports such as the Hospital Administrative Services (HAS) Report; some come from the cumulative experience of repeated applications of productivity measurement methodologies such as RMS; some come simply from the experiences of management engineering consultants who have dealt with the same kinds of tasks in a variety of institutional environments. Some specific examples include: 1.0 full-time equivalent (FTE) employee per one thousand discharges to staff a medical record department; 3.4 nursing hours per patient day to staff a routine medical/surgical nursing unit; 1.0 FTE per X-thousand square feet of floor space to staff a housekeeping department; 1.0 FTE per X-thousand annual admissions to staff an admitting department. The advantages of such guidelines, targets, and benchmarks are:

- They are quickly and inexpensively applied.
- Although crude they provide *some* standard, usually better than none at all.

The disadvantages of such indicators include:

- They are the least accurate of all performance standards used.
- Their applicability is always questionable. They represent the broadest of averages; they may be highly applicable in one setting and grossly inapplicable in another setting, and rarely will the user know which is the case in a particular institution.

HOW A PRODUCTIVITY STANDARD IS SET

A *productivity standard*—or a *time standard* or *work standard*, as it may also be called—is defined as the time required by a qualified and properly trained person working at a normal pace to do a specific task.[1] This standard may be expressed in terms of time per unit of work or in terms of work output per unit of time. The ultimate objective in using a time standard is to make possible an apples-to-apples comparison of output with input; since a standard allows output to be valued in terms of time, this amount of time may then be compared with the amount of time utilized as input.

Factors to Consider in Setting a Standard

In addition to the essential work content of a job, a number of additional factors will have a bearing on the manner in which the standard is set. The more significant factors include:

- The degree of repetitiveness of the task. A task that is performed only occasionally does not allow opportunity for the worker to get fully up to speed as would be the case with a task that is done over and over again. For many tasks, repetition builds familiarity which in turn builds output efficiency.
- The fatigue potential of the job. Some tasks, through either physical or mental demands, induce fatigue to an extent that can markedly affect performance time. Virtually all tasks induce fatigue to some degree: a person who enters a job fresh and rested is capable of greater performance than one who is tired from hours of work. This must be recognized in the time standards.
- Dependence on other employees. Many tasks are such that they cannot be completed alone; they require the accompanying efforts of other persons or they require related tasks to be accomplished first or perhaps between steps. This dependence, which is manifested in what may appear to be idle time, must be reflected in the time standard as long as it is valid.
- Interference. Natural disruptions sometimes prevent a worker from seeing a task through to completion, or work does not arrive in a time sequence that matches the worker's capacity. An interrupted task, one that must be stopped and restarted several times (such as the typing of a report by a secretary who doubles as a receptionist and thus must stop frequently to answer inquiries), will take longer because of the stops and starts than would otherwise be required. As to the timing of work arrival, a worker may be available to work but have nothing to do at times because no work has arrived. Some emergency room staffs experience interference factors in this respect; because of the essentially random arrival of patients they cannot always be gainfully occupied, but minimum staffing requirements dictate that a staff must always be there.

These and other factors, especially the methods employed in performing the task (see Chapter 8, Methods Improvement), are to be given whatever weight is necessary in setting the time standard.

THE GENERAL STANDARDS-SETTING PROCEDURE: ONE ILLUSTRATIVE METHOD

The supervisor (or management engineer or other work analyst) will ordinarily begin the process of setting productivity standards for a department by assessing the department's work and identifying all tasks that are done. Standards are most frequently established in order of the proportion of the department's time that various tasks require; that is, the first tasks for which standards are set are usually those that consume the largest part of the employees' time.

Assuming that a particular task has been identified and that a productivity standard is to be set, the process may proceed as follows:

1) The content of the task is analyzed for the purpose of identifying all steps involved, all inputs required, and all supporting activities that may have to take place for completion of the task. Special attention is given to identifying clearly recognizable starting and ending points for the task.

2) The content of every step is evaluated in detail, and every effort is made to alter the steps in the interest of improving productivity while not adversely affecting quality. Such evaluation will usually include attempts to reduce delays, reduce travel or handling, improve materials and equipment, and improve workplace layout (see Chapter 8).

3) Using one of the methods previously outlined—stopwatch time study, predetermined motion times, or work sampling—*normal time* for the task is determined. *Normal time* is the bare clock time, unaltered by allowances, for performing the task.

4) An appropriate factor is applied to compensate for personal, fatigue, and minor delay time that may be experienced. Commonly referred to as a PFD (personal, fatigue, and delay) factor, this may be established for the institution as a whole or for a specific department by extensive work-sampling study. Many hospitals use institution-wide PFD factors, most of which fall in the range of 15 to 20 percent. If the organization's PFD factor is 17 percent, for example, the normal time referred to in the preceding step is multiplied by 1.17 to arrive at the *standard time*, the time required by a qualified and properly trained person working at a normal pace to complete the task.

5) If not already accomplished, the department's *work units* should be clearly identified. These work units are the common units of service that constitute

the department's output, such as admissions (the admitting department), discharges (the medical record department), square feet of building space service (the housekeeping department), bills rendered (the patient billing function), tests (laboratory), procedures (radiology), meals served or patient days (food service).

6) Determine the *work unit time per occurrence* for each task. When such times for all tasks having a bearing on producing a unit of service are added together, the result will be *standard time per unit of service*.

7) It is next necessary to account for *indirect tasks* that are not accounted for in the standard thus far but nevertheless necessary to the production of the department's output. These can be handled in two ways.

- If there is a reasonable relationship between the indirect tasks and the units of service produced, that is, if the indirect work varies up or down as the units of service vary up or down, the indirect tasks (at least some of them) can be added to the standard as an additional per-unit allowance. For example, obtaining supplies, cleaning up after working, and preparing certain reports might be includable in the standard.
- If there is no direct relationship between indirect tasks and amount of output, indirect time may be expressed as an amount of constant time per day. Certain supporting activities, foremost among them supervision, secretarial support, and attending meetings, are departmental activities that occur to about the same extent regardless of variations in levels of output. For example, a given department may function at all times using one supervisor and one secretary over a broad range of output levels. Thus the resulting standard for an entire department is often a two-part expression—hours of constant time per day and time per unit of service.

8) The resulting *productivity standard* is applied in measuring and monitoring the department's productivity. Common forms of hospital productivity standards include:

- admitting: hours/calendar day, plus hours/admission;
- food service: hours/calendar day, plus hours/patient day;
- housekeeping: hours/calendar day (with staffing based on square feet of area);
- laboratory: hours/calendar day, plus hours/test; or, hours/calendar day, plus CAP units;
- medical records: hours/calendar day, plus hours/discharge;

- nursing (for specific nursing unit): hours/patient day;
- physical therapy: hours/calendar day, plus hours/modality.

9) It may at times be necessary to alter a department's productivity standard further to account for interference factors referred to earlier. Interference factors result from forces beyond the control of the supervisor, such as sporadic workload arrival, the need for standby coverage, and problems with physical layout. A *target utilization factor* may be established for this purpose. Usually based on a combination of measurement, observation, and judgment, a target utilization factor recognizes that practical productivity is often less than theoretical productivity. If a department's target utilization factor is 90 percent (an official recognition that 90 percent utilization is the maximum practical utilization for this department), the variable portion of the standard (the hours per unit of service) will be divided by 0.90 (inflated by ten percent) to reflect this. (The constant portion of the standard, the hours per calendar day, remains unadjusted.)

10) With or without the necessary adjustment of a target utilization factor, the *productivity standard* for a department will be of the form—usually two-part, but occasionally a single expression—described in step 8. This productivity standard makes it possible to value the department's output in terms of work time so output may be compared with work time applied as input.

EXAMPLE: HIGHLIGHTS OF THE PROCESS OF BUILDING A STANDARD FOR A DEPARTMENT

The department involved is the medical record department of a hospital. For consistency of discussion the ten steps appearing under the heading of *The Generalized Standards-Setting Procedure* are paralleled using the highlights of the process as actually applied in a particular medical record department.

1) All medical record tasks were clearly identified and listed. For this medical record department the task list consisted of:

- discharge processing, including coding, abstracting, and indexing;
- birth certificate processing;
- outpatient record processing;
- clinic patient record processing;
- emergency room record processing;
- telephone calls (incoming and outgoing);
- record pick up (from nursing units);

- information request processing (such as requests from insurance companies and attorneys);
- transcription;
- microfilming;
- filing;
- record assembly and analysis;
- review of incomplete records.

2) Every step of every task was evaluated for appropriateness of work methods, and changes were made where it appeared that work efficiency could be improved by doing so.

3) For every task listed above in number 1, a *normal time* was developed. For this medical record department normal times were developed using a combination of approaches (this is often the case). Special-purpose predetermined times, primarily from the RMS, were applied to most tasks. Some facets of microfilming and incomplete-record review were subjected to stopwatch time study. Time used on telephone calls and the processing of clinic and emergency room records were covered through a work sampling study. Once normal times were developed for all tasks, the times were extended by the amount of work activity experienced in a typical 4-week (28-day) period of representative activity. Work volume for the period was determined largely by actual count (primarily of actual discharges for the period); the frequency of some activities, notably telephone calls and filing, was established by direct survey of one period's activity. All extended times were summed to reveal that the variable tasks performed during the sample 4-week period should have required 951.23 *normal hours* to complete.

4) This medical record department (and in fact the entire hospital) used a PFD factor of 17 percent, inflating normal time accordingly: 951.23 hours × 1.17 = 1,112,93 standard hours.

5) The department's primary *work unit*, that is, the record department's principal unit of output, is the patient discharge. Although the department does some work that does not directly relate to the number of inpatient discharges, for example, processing of clinic records, enough of the department's total work is related to discharges to make this the primary variable. As the number of discharges varies, so also will the department's required work hours vary.

6) The *work unit time per occurrence* for this medical record department is:

$$\frac{1,112.93 \text{ standard hours}}{671 \text{ total discharges for the period}} = 1.659 \text{ variable hours/discharge.}$$

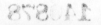

This is the *standard time per unit of service*. (This may also be arrived at by determining standard times for all individual tasks and adding them together. This would be done if standards were being developed for a few specific tasks or for part of the department only. Since the whole medical record department was being put on standard, however, it proved simpler to apply the PFD factor just once to the total and calculate standard time per occurrence once for the whole department rather than make these determinations separately for all tasks.)

7) The constant time (that time spent regardless of the volume of discharges) for a typical 4-week period amounted to:

- 400.0 hours of supervisory and secretarial time (one full-time supervisor and one full-time secretary);
- 18.7 hours of staff time devoted to special reports;
- 220.5 hours of staff time to operate the utilization review activity (reporting to medical records but excluded from standards determination).

Summed and distributed over the calendar days in the 4-week period, this amounts to 22.8 hours per day for *indirect* activities.

8) Combining the results of numbers 6 and 7, the *productivity standard* for this department is:

22.8 hours/calendar day + 1.659 hours/discharge.

9) A separate study revealed that approximately five percent of potential department productivity was lost because of the need to have a core staff present during the evenings. Thus the department's *target utilization* was established at 95 percent.

10) With target utilization factored in, the variable portion of the standard becomes:

$$\frac{1.659}{.95} = 1.746 \text{ hours per discharge.}$$

Thus the *productivity standard* becomes:

22.8 hours/calendar day + 1.746 hours/discharge.

As a productivity target this standard means that *on the average* (and it should always be stressed that standards are based on averages and as such are always subject to normal fluctuations) to operate this medical record department efficiently requires the expenditure of 22.8 hours in constant time every day plus 1.746 hours for every patient discharged from the hospital.

MONITORING DEPARTMENTAL PRODUCTIVITY

Productivity reporting for a department can be accomplished in a variety of ways depending on the specific kinds of information that management wishes to highlight. However, all productivity reporting uses as its basis the comparison of output produced with input consumed.

Exhibit 6-1 represents one common form of departmental productivity report. This example involves the medical record department described in the preceding section. Output in this report is valued according to the standard: 22.8 hours/calendar day + 1.746 hours/discharge. Reviewing the report column-by-column, from left to right:

Exhibit 6-1 Productivity Report: Medical Record Department
Standard: 22.8 hrs./day + 1.746 hrs./discharge

Period Ending	Volume (Discharges)		Worked Hours	Paid Hours	Worked FTEs				Paid FTEs			
	Budget	Actual			Req'd	Actual	Variance No.	Variance %	Budget	Actual	Variance No.	Variance %
1/26/85	671	642	1782	1996	11.0	11.1	0.1	1.0	13.5	12.5	(1.0)	(7.4)
2/23/85	671	668	1854	1965	11.3	11.6	0.3	2.7	13.5	12.3	(1.2)	(8.9)
3/23/85	671	690	1833	2053	11.5	11.5	0.0	0.0	13.5	12.8	(0.7)	(5.2)
4/20/85	671	676	1864	2013	11.4	11.6	0.2	1.8	13.5	12.6	(0.9)	(6.7)
Year to Date	2684	2676	7333	8027	11.3	11.5	0.2	1.8	13.5	12.5	(1.0)	(7.4)

FTE = full-time equivalent employee.
( ) = under budget.

Period Ending:

This is the date of the final day of the 4-week reporting period. (Productivity reports usually cover periods of two weeks, four weeks, or one month. Since payroll information is customarily kept in multiples of a week but operating statistics are often generated monthly, it is necessary to adjust one or the other. Ordinarily it is simpler to use a period consistent with payroll data and adjust the activity figures accordingly.)

Volume (Discharges):

Budget: From the hospital's statistical budget, this is the number of discharges projected to occur during the 4-week period. This may be the same for every period (as in this example) or it may vary if expected fluctuations have been accounted for in the budgeting process.

Actual: This is the number of discharges that actually occurred during the 4-week period.

Worked Hours:

This is the total number of hours that all medical record employees worked during the 4-week period.

Paid Hours:

This is the total hours paid to all medical record employees for the period, including all time actually worked (as reported under Worked Hours) plus all time-paid-not-worked, such as vacations, holidays, and paid sick time. Only straight-time hours are considered; that is, an hour's worth of overtime is reported as one paid hour although it may be compensated at time-and-one-half the appropriate hourly rate.

Worked FTEs:

Required: This is the number of FTEs that should be required to accomplish the department's work for the period, an expression of the amount of staff that should be *on hand and working* to meet the department's needs. It is arrived at by using the departmental standard to value the workload. For the period ending January 26, 1985, for example:

- 22.8 hours/day $\times$ 28 days + 1.746 hours/discharge $\times$ 642 discharges = 1,759.332 hours;
- 1.0 FTE = 40 hours/week $\times$ 4 weeks = 160 hours;
- $\dfrac{1759.332}{160}$ = 11.0 FTE.

Actual: This is the FTEs actually at work during the period, found by converting worked hours into FTEs. For the period ending January 26, 1985:

$$\frac{1782 \text{ worked hours}}{160 \text{ hours/FTE}} = 11.1 \text{ FTE}$$

Variance: The variance columns indicate the absolute number and the percentage by which actual staffing differs from required staffing. Actual staffing greater than required staffing yields a positive variance and thus an "overstaffed" situation (insignificant in the example).

Paid FTEs:
Budget: This column indicates the budgeted staffing level for the department. The sample suggests that this department is in the budget at a constant 13.5 FTEs, the product of a fixed budget (as opposed to a variable budget that might attempt to vary staffing—perhaps by varying part-time or optional staff—as workload might be projected to vary).

Actual: This is the medical record staff in FTEs actually paid for the period, including all time worked and all time-paid-not-worked. The number of FTEs paid will of course always be greater than the number of FTEs worked; there will always be the necessity to staff to allow for vacations, holidays, sick time, and other time-paid-not-worked.

Variance: The variance columns indicate where the department stands regarding FTEs actually paid as compared with FTEs allowed for in the budget. A negative (bracketed) variance indicates an underbudget situation.

Year to Date:
The year-to-date line contains summary calculations of all periods covered in the upper part of the report. Some comments that can be offered regarding the medical record department are:

- Actual workload has run extremely true to projections (2676 actual versus 2684 projected for the year to date).
- Actual staffing has been well in line with required staffing, showing only a +1.8 percent variance for 16 weeks. For most departments, a total year-to-date staffing variance within plus or minus five percent will be considered acceptable. Depending

on the particular department, the variance for any particular
4-week period may often vary as much as plus or minus ten percent with no action considered necessary as long as the year-to-
date variance remains within acceptable limits.

- The columns for *Paid FTEs* tell a slightly different story: Actual FTEs are running on the average one full FTE under budget
(variations in the numbers of the *Actual* column typically result
from using overtime or altering the hours of part-time
employees). It is likely that review of the details of the budget
would reveal that the department is carrying one position open
but unfilled. If this continues over most of the year, consideration should be given to removing from 0.5 to 1.0 FTE from the
next year's budget as long as projected activity appears to permit this.

As suggested, this example represents only one of several possible ways
of formatting and organizing a departmental productivity report. Regardless
of the specific approach used, however, the productivity report should provide constant visibility of the department's relationship between input and
output and should identify changes that are developing in that relationship.

WHO SHALL SET THE STANDARDS?

The supervisor can and should become well versed in productivity reporting and monitoring; as the maker of the department's resource allocation
decisions, he or she should have first-hand knowledge of how the department's human resources are being applied. However, for both practical and
technical reasons the supervisor may not be able to become totally immersed
in setting the standards.

Technically, the supervisor may not have or readily be able to acquire all
of the expertise necessary for setting standards. This chapter has included
some of the realm of the management engineer or industrial engineer, at least
from the supervisor's perspective, and yet has barely scratched the surface
of necessary engineering techniques. The supervisor may be able to apply
certain staffing guidelines with minimal technical background and also to
achieve competence in applying work sampling without spending a disproportionate amount of time learning this process. But learning to use the most
applicable work measurement techniques, notably the predetermined motion
time systems, specialized and otherwise, requires time that most supervisors
do not have.

This latter consideration—time—is the substance of the practical viewpoint
regarding the supervisor's involvement. Every supervisor is aware that it is

not possible to stop the clock and suspend all other activities while undertaking and completing a single major project. The development of a departmental standard is a major project, especially for an untrained analyst inexperienced in setting standards.

The persons best equipped to set the standards—hospital management engineers or management consultants—come from outside the department and often from outside the hospital. A person or persons experienced in setting work standards for health care activities should spearhead the effort. However, the supervisor and the employees, as persons left to live with the standards and make them work, should be active members of the standards team.

Numerous publications are available to the supervisor who wishes to gain some familiarity with techniques involved in establishing work standards. Listed below are three of the most comprehensive references available for information concerning the various techniques of work measurement. Within these three volumes interested readers will find references to dozens of additional sources of information. The basic references are:

- Ralph M. Barnes, *Motion and Time Study*, 7th ed. (New York: Wiley, 1980).
- H. B. Maynard, ed. *Industrial Engineering Handbook*, 3rd ed. (New York: McGraw-Hill, 1971).
- Harold E. Smalley, *Hospital Management Engineering: A Guide to Improvement of Hospital Management Systems* (Englewood Cliffs, N.J.: Prentice-Hall, 1982).

COST-EFFECTIVE STANDARDS SETTING

Despite the difficulty often involved in the process, with appropriate time and resources to apply in developing standards there remain few if any human activities that cannot be covered by reasonable standards. However, the selection of methods of setting standards should be based largely on cost effectiveness, that is, on the cost of application versus potential gains to be realized from the control of a particular activity.

An institution may apply a variety of approaches, using costly, time-consuming methods in areas of high activity and high cost and using crude guidelines in areas of minimal cost. A departmental standard may be set in much the same way, with major tasks covered by in-depth analysis and small, infrequent tasks valued by using guidelines and estimates based on observation.

Reasonable standards and a productivity monitoring system are only the beginning. Control, one of the supervisor's basic management functions, consists of information *and action*. Standards and the monitoring system provide the information; the supervisor must act on that information to maintain output in an efficient relationship to input.

NOTE

1. Ralph M. Barnes, *Motion and Time Study*, 6th ed. (New York: Wiley, 1968), p. 4.

The Human Factor

It is people that count; you want to put yourself into people; they touch other people; these others still; and so you go on working forever.

Alice Freeman Palmer

Chapter Objectives

- Place the human worker in proper perspective as the critical variable in determining productivity.
- Review the basic human needs that provide the motivation to work.
- Review the expectations that employees place on their work organizations.
- Outline the various facets of the supervisor's role in the fulfillment of employee needs.
- Explore the apparent relationship between employee training and productivity.

HUMAN RELATIONS AND PRODUCTIVITY

The Critical Variable

A young but accomplished short-order cook decided to go into the restaurant business on his own. He started in a small way by opening a diner that was strictly a one-person operation. He quickly learned that because of his location relative to several businesses, the breakfast period was his busiest time of day. He knew he had to be efficient and highly productive because he was working alone; he sensibly arranged his major work area around him so that he could reach everything needed with minimum movement and could fill orders at maximum possible speed. He became extremely adept at placing complete appealing meals before the customers at the counter just minutes after the orders were given.

The diner operator was so successful that he was able to expand his establishment and add some booths and tables. He decided he would have more flexibility if he worked as manager, waiter, and cashier, so he advertised for an experienced short-order cook. He put the new cook to work, and the cook's first day was a disaster.

It is not unusual for one's first day on a new job to be less than outstanding. However, day one became day two, then day three—the first full week had passed and the new cook was still wallowing in disaster. Some customers were complaining; some were simply not returning. Eggs were being dropped, coffee and juice were being spilled, toast was being burned, and orders were being mixed up and served cold. Where the proprietor had formerly been a model of speed, efficiency, and quality, the new cook—who basically was as good a cook as the proprietor had been—was falling all over himself, breaking things, and generally destroying the business.

After one week of disappointment and dismay, the cause of the new cook's apparent ineptness became clear to the proprietor: the new cook was left-handed. He, the proprietor, was right-handed and had set up his highly efficient work area to suit himself.

After one additional day's observation (extremely fruitful, because now the proprietor knew what he was looking for) the proprietor developed a plan for a new workplace layout. In a single evening and with the outlay of a few dollars for material, he rearranged the work area to accommodate the special requirements of the left-handed cook. Within one working day the cook accomplished a complete turnabout in performance and the problem was solved.

The point of the story is: *There is no such thing as a standard person.* Each person is different from everyone else in a number of ways, and most differences are subtler than the modest physiological difference of being left-handed in a largely right-handed world. Not everyone fits the same way into every situation, and the realization that this is so should lead management to appreciate that productivity depends not only on what is done with the job but also on what is done with and for the human being who performs the job.

Health care managers are inclined to regard health care as totally different from all other endeavors; in many ways it is vastly different from most other activities. However, in one important respect health care is precisely the same as all others: work is done by people. As Rensis Likert in *New Patterns of Management* says, "The end product of all business is people."[1] All providers of products or services work *with* people and *for* people and must please people in order to survive over the long run.

Recall the frequently cited Hawthorne experiment of 1927 to 1932. This was a large-scale, controlled experiment in which job factors in a manufacturing setting were varied, generally toward improvement, and changes in employee productivity were noted. For a time there was a direct relationship between working conditions and productivity; as conditions were continually improved, productivity continued to increase. However, when some conditions in the work environment were deliberately made less desirable (at one time, for example, the number of allowed breaks was reduced), *productivity still continued to increase.*[2]

Why did workers continue to increase output even as working conditions were made supposedly less desirable? The researchers concluded that this occurred because someone was paying attention to the workers. To quote a passage from one of the Hawthorne study reports:

> There has been a continual upward trend in output which has
> been independent of the changes in rest pauses. This upward trend
> has continued too long to be ascribed to an initial stimulus from
> the novelty of starting a special study.[3]

It is now generally accepted that the significant factors influencing productivity center about the workplace and its social nature even more than about the physical factors affecting the job. To some extent workers' mental attitudes are shaped by the work situation, and to some extent these attitudes are also influenced by patterns of behavior brought onto the job from outside of the organization. In other words, refined work methods and scientifically engineered work stations, although important in their own right, are often the lesser stimulants of improved productivity; it is usually the physiological, intellectual, and emotional state of the workers that must be reckoned with as the larger collection of stimuli for improved productivity. Thus it is these latter characteristics, and especially the emotional and intellectual factors, which the supervisor must address with the employee to stimulate improved productivity. An unhappy or dissatisfied employee is probably not producing up to full potential. The relationship of productivity to employee relations is clear; the better the leadership that is provided, the more likely the employee is to be satisfied. The more satisfied the employee, the more productive that employee is likely to be.

Despite all the attention that can and should be given to the engineering and business aspects of the enhancement of productivity—correct materials and supplies, proper equipment, sound workplace layout, and appropriate logistics and support—the human worker remains the most critical and yet the least predictable variable in determining productivity.

DEALING WITH THE HUMAN VARIABLE

One could write a volume, perhaps even several volumes, about human relations in supervision, and do so without exhausting the subject. Instead of repeating theory and proven practical advice that are available in other books, however, we will present a number of reminders of the determinants of appropriate supervisory behavior. These few reminders will be based on the supervisor's role in the fulfillment of the needs of employees as members of a work organization.

The starting premise of this discussion, alluded to earlier, is that the employee who is generally satisfied with most major dimensions of the work relationship is likely to be more productive and more cooperative than the employee who is dissatisfied. This is not to suggest, however, that it is realistic for one to expect to guarantee the complete satisfaction of all employees with all aspects of the work relationship. Each person is vastly different from each other person; many will be satisfied and thus productive if dealt with fairly and squarely by the supervisor and the organization; some will never be totally satisfied no matter what is done to please them. Under the proper conditions many people enjoy work, but there are some (a minority, one would hope, but by nature troublesome to the supervisor) who simply do not enjoy work or who at least do not care for the kinds of work they do out of economic necessity.

One should never be led, even by default, that is, by not thinking about it, to believe that it is possible to create conditions conducive to employee satisfaction and then let the business of human relations take care of itself. One of the many corollaries of the well-known *Murphy's Law* suggests: *Left unto themselves, things invariably go from bad to worse.* It is true that the establishment of an open, honest, effective one-to-one relationship with each employee is an important task of the supervisor. However, an even more important task, much more important because it is ongoing, is the supervisor's maintenance of each such relationship.

Most supervisors can do a great deal to enhance the productivity of a work group through effective human relations. The task often looms large; unfortunately, traditional organizations have built in a fair amount of dissatisfaction at all organizational levels. So much work has been structured, subdivided, and systematized that human factors beyond mere job performance are ignored and the inherent challenge of work as a normal human activity is diluted or dissipated. People respond to work in terms of personal needs and desires, so productive efficiency turns out to be not especially satisfying in itself. Management must seek ways and means of allowing employees to satisfy basic personal needs through work.

Basic Human Needs: Maslow Revisited

Each employee will achieve some level of personal satisfaction according to how well a unique collection of needs may be met. In his well-known "need hierarchy," A. H. Maslow described the basic human needs as follows:[4]

- Physiological needs are the most fundamental—the things required to sustain life, such as food and shelter.
- Safety needs include the need to feel reasonably free from harm from others and to feel reasonably free from economic deprivation (this is reflected, for example, in the need for job security).
- Love needs include the need to be liked by others and to be accepted as part of a group, be it a work, family, or social group. Needs at this level involve a sense of belonging.
- Esteem needs are needs for recognition, for approval, for assurance that what one is doing is appreciated.
- Self-actualization needs represent "a pressure toward unity of personality, toward being creative, toward being good, and a lot else."

Maslow suggests that all people proceed through the need hierarchy from the most fundamental needs toward needs of the highest order. Once a need is satisfied, another arises to take its place, and thus a person experiences needs of increasingly higher order. For those in need of food, clothing, and shelter, basic physiological and safety needs motivate their behavior. Regarding work and these needs, a person with unmet physiological and safety needs will not likely be spurred onward by the lure of interesting work experiences or appreciation of accomplishments. At that level a person is most interested in generating an income with which to buy the basics of life.

However, once these lower order needs have been satisfied to a reasonable extent, one begins to experience the love needs, to look for acceptance, and to attempt to secure membership in various groups. Thus one progresses through the hierarchy until ultimately motivated by the need for self-actualization.

The need hierarchy has been rather firmly established, but there are vast differences among people as to individual needs and thus corresponding differences in what is required to satisfy those needs. For instance, one person's need for assurance of reasonable job security may be filled by the knowledge that the job will last at least another three months, while another person may feel uneasy unless assured the job will last until retirement. Also, love needs and esteem needs may be powerful in an individual who requires constant reassurance of worth and capability, while another person may experience fewer needs at this level simply because of the presence of a high degree of self-confidence and sense of self-worth. Regardless, however, of the needs actually experienced by any particular individual, the matter of progression through the need hierarchy holds true: As a need is reasonably satisfied, another higher order need arises to take its place.

People have vastly different reasons for working. As in this country formerly, today in some underdeveloped countries people concentrate most of their energies simply on remaining fed, clothed, and sheltered at a minimal level; they rarely go beyond the level of physiological and safety needs. In modern industrial society, however, lower order needs are satisfied for many people most of the time. People experience higher order needs and proceed to seek satisfaction. Even the person who feels continually driven by the same goal, for instance, money, will be doing so for changing reasons. Once reasonable economic security is no longer a concern, money may be seen as the means of securing leisure time, social acceptabilty, status, prestige, and perhaps even power and influence, all expressions of higher order needs.[5]

Demands on the Organization

People want the organization for which they work to supply a certain number of things. Since that which is important to some person may matter little to another, these items cannot be listed in any specific order of importance. Generally, however, one should find that the following list encompasses most of what employees expect of their employers:

- capable leadership that can be respected and admired;
- decent working conditions: surroundings that promote safety and physical well-being;
- acceptance as a member of a group;

- recognition as an individual or partner, not simply as a servant of the system;
- fair treatment relative to that received by others;
- a reasonable degree of job security;
- knowledge of the results of individual efforts;
- knowledge of the organization's policies, rules, and regulations;
- recognition for special effort or good performance;
- respect for individual religious, moral, and political beliefs;
- assurance that all others are doing their share of the work;
- fair monetary compensation.[6]

The Supervisor's Role in Satisfaction of Employee Needs

It must be recognized that the "demands" employees place on the organization will vary greatly according to individuals' needs. The foregoing list of demands encompasses human needs from throughout the hierarchy. For example, the desire for job security largely reflects safety needs; acceptance as a member of a group fulfills love needs; knowledge of the results of individual efforts and recognition for special effort or good performance reflect esteem needs.

Because of the nature of the supervisory position and the organizational authority vested in that position, the supervisor is able to control employees' fulfillment of certain needs and at least to influence to some extent the fulfillment of other needs. With respect to a number of employee needs the supervisor is even able to control fulfillment by providing or withholding need satisfaction at will (although to withhold need satisfaction consciously for reasons of controlling employees is clearly manipulative).

Following is a brief recounting of the supervisor's role relative to employee needs, with special attention given to the extent of the supervisor's ability to control need satisfaction. This listing parallels "Demands on the Organization."

1) *Leadership*. A great deal can be said about what a leader should be, what a leader should do, and how an effective leader is to be characterized. Who can say, at least without extensive study, that employees follow a supervisor because of the supervisor's leadership capability or simply because of the organizational authority of the supervisory position? In the end the single factor that defines or characterizes a true leader is acceptance of the followers. This acceptance cannot be mandated; it must be earned. Without such acceptance a supervisor is a supervisor by title only, and not at all a leader. The employee's need for capable leadership that can be respected and ad-

mired is one for which fulfillment lies completely in the hands of the supervisor. In brief, the successful leader will be one who:

- communicates openly, sharing all necessary or helpful information with the employee group;
- displays awareness of employees' problems and needs;
- displays trust and confidence in the employees;
- motivates employees by positive means, through involvement and reward;
- provides support to employees, letting them know that they do not stand alone when things go wrong;
- requests input from employees whenever possible, recognizing that each employee is capable of contributing something;
- consistently treats all employees fairly and equally.

2) *Working conditions.* The supervisor may not always, indeed may never, be able to control working conditions directly. For the most part the temperature of the office, the state of the heating and air conditioning, the quality of the cafeteria food, the condition of the parking lot, and many other factors may lie beyond the supervisor's immediate control. However, the supervisor can and should be a monitor of working conditions, should listen to employees and, if convinced that something does need to be changed or improved, become the employees' advocate in working with other parts of the organization to do so. The message conveyed by the supervisor's action should be clear: "I care about your safety, comfort, and well-being on the job, and I want to help you do your work by providing the best possible environment in which to work."

3) *Acceptance.* The supervisor has much control over the acceptance of the individual employee as a member of the work group. The supervisor should be the person who takes the lead in making a new employee feel welcome to the departmental team. Each employee should feel that full group membership is extended to every employee equally. There are of course numerous groups that can form within the work setting, and the supervisor cannot control membership in all of them—for example, friendships in varying degrees of closeness will be present—but the supervisor can at least see that each employee is given an equal chance to be an integral part of the work group. Beyond the formal work group, through careful assignment of work the supervisor can discourage the formation and perpetuation of cliques that may tend to exclude people from membership either actively or passively.

4) *Recognition as an individual or partner.* An employee's immediate supervisor controls recognition in two ways. The first lies in basic human relations, in the supervisor's recognition of each employee as an individual having rights, needs, and feelings and deserving equal opportunity to earn the respect of others in the organization. The second involves the supervisor's continuing efforts to assure employees that they are part of a team and that their contributions matter or they would not be there.

5) *Fair treatment.* The supervisor has a lot of control regarding individual employee fair treatment relative to treatment of others. The key word in the preceding sentence is *relative*. There may be times when the treatment of members of the work group may not be perceived as fair when judged by some personal standard—for example, many people may think it unfair to have all the staff of an empty nursing unit take leave without pay because there are no patients and thus no revenue—but within the group the treatment can be fair if applied equally to all. In other words it is usually not the absolute treatment of an employee that matters nearly as much as how that employee is treated relative to the way others are treated. The supervisor should avoid playing favorites and should avoid actions that may convey the appearance of favoritism.

6) *Job security.* Often the supervisor has little control over job security; after all, the individual supervisor has no control over business conditions that govern the continued employment of the organization's workers. However, the supervisor can avoid using fears about job security as a misdirected motivator. Occasional supervisors, usually those with authoritarian leanings, unconsciously (and sometimes consciously) practice motivation by fear, allowing employees to believe that the rule is "one slip and you're out." While a healthy desire to remain employed is a legitimate motivator inspiring one to continue performing, it can become unhealthy if this desire is created by the fear of termination. Fearful persons are rarely capable of doing their best. Generally the best work comes from those employees who are encouraged to contribute, are allowed to be innovative, and know that they have the freedom to fail occasionally.

7) *Knowledge of the results of individual efforts.* The degree of supervisory influence in this case will generally vary with the kinds of work being done. The purchasing agent who negotiates a particularly good deal can immediately see the results of his efforts; the nurse who calms a distraught patient can immediately see the results of her efforts. But much work is such that the worker cannot see the outcome. The cook, for example, does not know whether the patient liked the meal; the billing clerk does not know what dif-

ference today's billings, so carefully prepared and reconciled, may make in the state of the institution's business. The work is not always such that the supervisor can assure the employees' knowledge of the results of their efforts. There are, however, two important things the supervisor can do: solicit and otherwise secure feedback for employees regarding the results of their efforts; and practice proper delegation in such a way that employees regularly handle whole tasks from start to finish where possible—not just bits and chunks—so they can view at least part of the job with a sense of completeness.

8) *Knowledge of policies, rules, and regulations.* In this extremely important area of employee communication the supervisor has almost total control. The supervisor should be the employee's primary source of information about how the organization does things and what is expected in employee conduct. It is the supervisor's responsibility to assure that each employee is aware of all pertinent work rules and policies. This responsibility is fulfilled through comprehensive orientation to both institution and department, by answering employees' questions and supplying policy interpretations when the need arises, and by actively seeking answers and clarifications needed by employees for which the supervisor cannot provide immediate responses. The supervisor who assures that the employees' knowledge of policies, rules, and regulations is as complete as possible, and assures that questions the supervisor cannot answer are researched and answered in timely fashion, can minimize or eliminate numerous possible unknowns that could otherwise add to employee dissatisfaction.

9) *Recognition for special effort or good performance.* Here the supervisor can exert total control. It is easy for the harried, overworked supervisor to take special effort or good performance for granted, perhaps in the unconscious belief that no response is required or that successful performance is its own reward. Successful performance may indeed be its own reward for a few employees, but most people need some degree of continuing assurance that they are doing well. The employee who receives no feedback on performance except perhaps during the annual appraisal works long periods not knowing how performance is viewed. The employee who receives no feedback often experiences doubts; lack of response could mean that performance has been taken as anything from marginally acceptable (barely missing criticism) to outstanding. The supervisor who regularly praises special effort or good performance can do much to reduce employees' feelings of uncertainty that can lead to dissatisfaction. Most employees need to know where they stand in the eyes of the supervisor most of the time.

10) *Respect.* One might respond to the call for respect by suggesting that respect is earned. This is certainly true as regards respect for an individual

arising from attitude and conduct—respect arising from displays of honesty, energy, cooperation, and so on. In this regard each employee must earn the respect of bosses and co-workers alike. Regarding an individual's religious, moral, and political beliefs, however, each employee needs and is legally entitled to under Equal Employment Opportunity consideration and treatment equal to that extended to all other employees. The supervisor must take the lead in extending this treatment, and further, the supervisor must assure that co-workers do not discriminate against those whose beliefs are in the minority in the work group.

11) *Assurance that all others are doing their share of the work.* Like item 5, which is concerned with fair treatment relative to that received by others, many employees need continuing assurance that all persons in the work group are pulling their weight equally. Few conditions are more likely to cause employee dissatisfaction than when some employees are obviously carrying others who are not doing their expected share. It is up to the supervisor to assure, given the department's mix of skills, talents, and capabilities, that each employee is earning his or her own way through acceptable performance (which includes acceptable quantity of output). The supervisor must do so through conscientious attention to job content and work assignments, and through disciplining and otherwise working with apparent slackers or substandard performers. The generally satisfied work group is one which the members are able to feel like a team of equal contributors. Even if the group as a whole should happen to feel overworked or overburdened, dissatisfaction can be minimized if the group's employees can view each other in a way that suggests they believe "we're all in this together."

12) *Monetary compensation.* The supervisor ordinarily has no control over the levels of wages paid for various skills in the department. However, depending on the system of setting hiring rates and granting increases, the supervisor may have some influence on the way the wage and salary system is administered. Employees will of course have widely varying notions of what constitutes fair monetary compensation; certainly few employees would ever refuse to accept more money for doing the work they perform. Fairness will be a perception based in part on what others in the community and organization are receiving for the same kind of work; this perception will often include beliefs in reward for loyalty (seniority or longevity) and beliefs in reward for performance (merit pay). As suggested, most of the major elements of the wage and salary system will lie beyond the individual supervisor's control, but the supervisor can practice strict fairness in applying those elements of the system that can be controlled at department level and report pay inequities, both real and perceived, to higher management so these can be investigated

and acted upon as necessary. With pay, as with so many other elements of the employment relationship, one of the key considerations is fairness relative to others.

RELATIONSHIP BETWEEN TRAINING AND PRODUCTIVITY

Most managers will agree that there is a positive relationship between appropriate training and productivity, that training can and often does stimulate both managers and nonmanagers to improve their productivity. However, there appears to be little general agreement on how the impact of training on productivity can be measured or whether it can be measured at all. Yet it was recognized a number of years ago by the National Commission on Productivity and Work Quality that one of the conditions required for improved productivity within the health care industry was "increased knowledge and skill of the work force."[7]

It is necessary to differentiate between consideration of training for nonmanagerial employees and education of managers, or at least to differentiate between knowledge and skill training versus the nurturing of attitudes.

Many employees come to the health care institution already reasonably well trained, some arrive partly trained, and some arrive having had no training at all. For such untrained or partly trained employees, especially those who are not managers, the institution's training task is usually to:

- teach specific skills and techniques either in a formal setting or through on-the-job training or some combination thereof;
- teach the institution's specific methods and operating procedures;
- maintain or upgrade skills, and provide refresher training.

Once a normally expected level of productivity is attained, however, skill-and-knowledge training swiftly approaches a point of diminishing returns. Thus we suggest that perhaps most worker education beyond skill-and-knowledge training should focus on attitudes, with the recognition that improving productivity or even maintaining acceptable levels of productivity depends more on motivation than on skill and knowledge. In short, the employee should eventually strive to accomplish more because of a personal desire to do so.

Continuing education programs and ongoing worker information programs used to supplement an overall effective employee relations program can be intuitively accepted as having the potential to increase productivity. Management needs eventually to recognize that one cannot really motivate an employee but can only create the climate in which the worker will become self-motivated.

Problems of measurement remain, however. Except for examinations administered to sample the results of skill-and-knowledge programs, most training program evaluations are highly subjective. To be successful in measuring the results of most educational programs, one must observe the before-and-after behavior of the trainees and determine whether there has been any substantive change in behavior. Because of the impracticability of measuring program results through observations of behavior, most evaluations fall back on subjective techniques usually including the use of questionnaires to sample the reactions and opinions of attendees. Few quantitative measures are available, and most that are available are technically sophisticated and costlier to use than the training program they would attempt to assess. Even so-called objective examinations following skill-and-knowledge programs reveal only temporary retention of factual information. They say nothing at all about altered behavior.

The supervisor must intuitively accept the belief that the positive productivity-related benefits of employee training are there, and that despite the lack of objective measurements it is less costly to train than not to train. For example, who can positively identify the value of the benefit accruing to the organization because:

- an expensive piece of equipment was *not* lost because its operator had received proper training?
- a malpractice suit was avoided because an employee was knowledgeable of the potential consequences of her actions?
- a possible unfair labor practice charge was avoided because a supervisor knew his limitations under the Fair Labor Standards Act?
- a budget did not have to be completely reworked because a manager was skilled in budgeting techniques?
- any conceivable error was avoided because an employee had been properly educated?

Supervisory Development

Any discussion of the relationship between productivity and training would be incomplete without some attention to the development of supervisory skills. Supervisory skill development is widespread within health care institutions for good reason—the supervisor is in a position to influence the productivity of every employee in the work group. The direct impact of most supervisory development, however, is unmeasurable, but one must believe that it nevertheless exists.

The attitude toward supervisory development requires a balanced perspective. It is a mistake to believe that two dozen supervisors who sit through a few two-hour training sessions will then go forth and set the managerial world on fire. Rather, a healthy curiosity aroused in two or three of two dozen attendees—a curiosity that will remain and may surface through future action—can mean resounding success for a supervisory skills development program. A program can be considered a success if, sometime during the weeks and months following its conclusion, two or three supervisors are led to think something like: "We talked about this kind of situation in one of those classes. I'm going to try to apply what I remember and see if it works."

One of the most important things that many supervisors have to learn is that *they really are supervisors*. Many came into their positions by advancement from technical specialties. In all probability they had years of specialized training within their chosen fields, but their entry into management was probably by appointment and accomplished with no training in supervisory skills.

Complete lack of management education notwithstanding, it is likely that most new supervisors have considerable knowledge of what managers are supposed to know and do. Thus, supervisory skills development should not be intended primarily to implant knowledge that will be applied later but should nurture the attitudes necessary to make supervisors think of themselves as true managers—to think like managers and to act like managers.

Methods Improvement Training

In view of a need for renewed, continuing emphasis on productivity, one form of employee education, equally applicable to managers and nonmanagers alike, is especially valuable: training in the specific techniques of methods improvement or work simplification. A model health care employee training program for the coming several years might be one that focuses on the techniques of cost reduction and work simplification using real-life problems taken from the work situations of the program attendees.

One example: A small group of hospitals commissioned the development of a methods improvement program for six groups of employees. Each class, consisting of 20 to 25 people, was subdivided into project groups of four to five people each. Each attendee was expected to bring in a job-related problem of some apparent cost reduction potential. Each project group screened the four or five projects supplied by its members and selected the potentially most productive one to work on. In total, the members of the six classes pursued 30 methods improvement projects.

After several weeks' activity during which the classes met formally for a half-day each week and the project groups met as they were able and needed to do so, 30 project reports were presented. Nearly half of the 30 projects revealed potential dollar savings, and all 30 projects offered significant tangible benefits. In summary:

- One project revealed ongoing savings of $10,000 to $15,000 per year, available for a total implementation cost of less than $1,000.
- One project offered avoidance of an approved and supposedly inevitable expenditure of $6,000, and did so with no out-of-pocket expense.
- Several other projects offered annually recurring savings, net of implementation costs, of $9,000, $6,000, $4,000, and $2,000 respectively.
- Overall the projects identified potential net annual savings of approximately $44,000 per year.

The total cost of providing the methods improvement program for the six classes was approximately $6,000. It was felt that a $6,000 one-time expenditure for an annually recurring return of $44,000 was a bargain. Thus, budget-conscious management which has problems accepting the cost of education and looks for measurable returns might wish to consider a cost reduction and methods improvement program using actual problems taken from the participants' jobs.

Methods improvement programs aside, however, it remains difficult to measure the effects of employee education. Management can see and count the scarce dollars that must be spent to purchase educational programs and material, hire trainers, and engage educational consultants; these are recognizable expenditures. However, it is not as easy to see the money leaking through the cracks because an institution has no concrete program to help employees approach their productive potential.

At a time when health care institutions need the best efforts their employees can give, they cannot afford to fail to emphasize education. As Henry Ford is credited with saying, "Education is not something to prepare you for life; it is a continuous part of life."

NOTES

1. Rensis Likert, *New Patterns of Management* (New York: McGraw-Hill, 1961).
2. Elton Mayo, *The Human Problems of an Industrial Civilization* (New York: Viking Press, 1960), pp. 65–67.
3. Ibid.
4. A.H. Maslow, "A Theory of Human Motivation," *Psychological Review* 50 (1943): 370–396.
5. Portions of "Basic Human Needs: Maslow Revisited" were adapted from Charles R. McConnell, *The Effective Health Care Supervisor* (Rockville, Md.: Aspen Systems Corp., 1982), Chap. 11, "Motivation: Intangible Forces and Slippery Rules."
6. McConnell, *The Effective Health Care Supervisor*, p. 117.
7. National Commission on Productivity and Work Quality, *Report of the Hospital and Health Care Committee* (Washington, D.C.: GPO, 1975).

Chapter 8

Methods Improvement*

I keep six honest serving men,
(They taught me all I know);
Their names are what and why and where
And how and when and who.

Rudyard Kipling

Chapter Objectives

- Convey the belief that there is usually room for improvement in the way most tasks are performed.
- Outline a simple, logical approach to improvement of work methods.
- Introduce some of the more common tools and techniques of methods improvement and provide guidelines for their application.
- Outline an organized approach to methods improvement applicable institution-wide.
- Identify the role of the supervisor in encouraging a "methods-minded attitude" on the part of the department's employees.

---

*Portions of this chapter were adapted from Charles R. McConnell, *The Effective Health Care Supervisor* (Rockville, Md.: Aspen Systems Corp., 1982), pp. 249–263.

EDISON-PLUS

Thomas A. Edison is credited with saying, "There's a way to do it better—find it." There is no hedging in Edison's statement, no qualifier that might keep the door to improvement closed. Edison did not say there is sometimes, often, or even usually a better way, just there *is* a better way. Often there are several better ways.

Some pioneers of industrial engineering, the branch of engineering dealing with work methods, insisted on the need to seek something they referred to as the *one best way*. In recent years, however, the notion of a single best way to do a job is regarded as a theoretical ideal. It is now recognized that there are usually several better ways of accomplishing a task and that it is necessary to seek one of these better ways that reasonably meets the needs of the situation and fulfills the objectives of the organization.

Methods improvement can be described as the organized approach to determining how to accomplish a task with less effort, in less time, or at lower cost, while maintaining or improving the quality of the outcome. This process may also be referred to in different organizations by various other labels, among them *methods engineering, job improvement,* and *work simplification*. Regardless of label, however, the intent is the same: to alter the performance of a task in such a way that the results represent a desired improvement.

Methods improvement is understandably a subject that is not near and dear to a great many supervisors. Rarely is the need for change in a specific work procedure so pressing that it takes priority over the day-to-day, hour-to-hour operating problems of a department. However, methods improvement is one management activity that puts supervisors in a bind—rarely is it critical and it is usually freely postponable, but unless it is made part of today's effort the department will never realize its near-future benefits. Much like delegation, it is an activity we promise to take seriously "after the rush is over," but we never quite get around to it.

A modest but active methods improvement program can be a valuable part of any supervisor's pattern of management. Economic benefits can be gained: When a job is accomplished in less time, with less effort, or with fewer material resources, the relationship between output and input is bettered and the department's efficiency is improved. There are also less tangible benefits to consider. When methods improvement is approached with a spirit of participative management, and uses the contributions of people who actually do the work, there are positive returns in employee attitude.

ROOM FOR IMPROVEMENT

Methods improvement may exist as a formal program in the organization, coordinated by a department such as management engineering or industrial engineering or management systems. Or it may exist at the department level, at the discretion of the supervisor, as an informal, ongoing effort to tune up and otherwise improve work procedures. At the least, methods improvement should exist in the department as an attitude. Such a methods-minded attitude, a practiced belief in the possibility of continuing improvement, will itself encourage employees to use time and other resources more effectively.

Methods improvement applies largely to tasks, to problems of things (such as procedures, processes, forms, equipment, and physical layout) as opposed to problems of people. It is generally recognized that the task of getting things done through people puts the supervisor in a position of being largely a solver of people problems. However, it must also be recognized that work procedures and other nonhuman factors are nevertheless shaped or influenced by the people who do the work. A certain procedure may lose efficiency over months or years because of the changing environment in which the job is performed, but efficiency may also be lost because people bring their own habits, attitudes, and preferences onto the job, which influences the way they work. Dig deeply enough into causes and one will often find that many seemingly nonpeople problems have human origins.

Each person coming to work in the department is a unique individual and exerts a unique influence on the workplace. Thus a work procedure, especially one not well defined previously, becomes in part a reflection of the worker. When several consecutive individuals have been assigned in turn to the same specific task, the result—how that task is done today—is often a composite procedure that incorporates the subtle and not-so-subtle influences of these several people. Since many employees are trained on the job using the example of the person actually doing the job, not only essential job knowledge but also influences of other workers are passed along.

A procedure for performing a given task may exist in a department in three different ways. It can exist in one form in the mind of the supervisor who, perhaps having done the job at one time, thinks of a specific (and quite likely outdated) collection of steps. The procedure can also exist in the mind of the worker in the form of all the steps this person actually performs to accomplish the task. It may also exist in writing in the department's procedure manual in a form different from either the supervisor's concept or the worker's practice; and how often are such manuals referred to when people believe that the same old task is being done in the same old way?

In some organizations, concern for methods improvement is left to a specific group such as management engineering. However, the power to improve procedures and make work easier need not be limited to some special staff. A simple philosophy of methods improvement, readily put into practice at the department level, might suggest the following:

- There are few, if any, existing tasks that cannot be improved.
- The people who actually do the work are potentially valuable contributors to improvement.
- The power of participative management can bring out the best in each employee.

From a healthy, participative management point of view, methods improvement may be simply described as *applied common sense*.

THE METHODS IMPROVEMENT APPROACH

A generalized several-step approach to methods improvement will be presented, following which some of the simpler tools and techniques of methods analysis will be reviewed. Successful methods improvement ordinarily begins with concentration on a single, specific task. A supervisor has too much to do to attempt to make everything better at once; a "shotgun" approach will lead to the start of many projects but the likely completion of few or none. Select one task or isolate one problem (something that is creating trouble or something that some workers feel could be done more efficiently) and go to work.

Select a Task or Isolate a Problem

It is necessary first to become aware of a problem before it can be solved. The need for methods improvement will often become apparent on a number of fronts if the several areas in which the department's problems usually arise are examined in detail. The significant signs that often suggest that a particular task deserves analysis and improvement are:

- An activity is costing more to perform than is generally known or believed that it should cost.
- Bottlenecks occur as work backs up at various stages of a process, or there are chronic backlogs of incomplete work.
- Confusion is evident as employees appear uncertain as to what happens next, how it happens, and why.

- Poor morale prevails in the work group, or there is a noticeable pattern of worker grievances and complaints related to modes of work performance.
- Walking, handling, transportation, and other nonproductive activities appear to occur in excess.

In locating and defining problems which may highlight the need for methods improvement, it is important to distinguish between problem symptoms and true causal problems. For example, that which might appear to be a bottleneck caused by poor working methods might seem to be readily corrected by applying a small amount of overtime, a bit of extra effort, or a rearrangement in task assignments. However, if the true causal problem lies in ineffective scheduling practices, the bottleneck, supposedly fixed, is likely to return once conditions revert to normal. When that which is addressed head on is in reality a symptom of a problem, the difficulty will likely return within a short time or resurface in altered form. Thus it is necessary to look beyond the apparent immediate problem and identify the force or forces that lie behind this manifestation of difficulty.

Gather the Facts

It is necessary to learn thoroughly how a task is done now, to learn everything one can possibly learn about the way the job is being performed. By using sketches or flowcharts or whatever other techniques are available, the total process involved in the task under consideration must be described. Sketching out the system often aids in increasing understanding of the relationships that exist among system components, since a logical order or reasonable interrelationship of pieces can often be observed once the components are all captured on paper. Further, recording the present method in full also allows others who can provide insight into the problem to examine the process and compare it with their understanding of the situation.

In getting the facts—in applying the information-gathering tools and techniques of methods improvement—one may gather information from:

- written procedures, if such already exist in some form;
- architectural and layout drawings, if the problem concerns workplace layout or physical space in any way;
- work schedules;
- samples of pertinent forms and records;
- accounting data, payroll data, purchasing information, budgets, and other financial records;
- statistical reports and other records of operating results.

One may be sure, however, that what is collected through any of the foregoing sources will often not be sufficient. It is usually necessary to expend additional effort on the one major area of concern that cannot be learned about from existing information: *how the task is currently being performed.*

Reduce the Problem to Sub-Problems as Necessary

Often a single apparent methods improvement problem may appear to be too large or too complex to tackle as a whole. However, such a problem can often be broken down into a number of smaller, separately identifiable problems that can be solved largely independently of each other. A number of difficulties may have shown up in a regularly recurring backlog of medical record transcription and come together in what appears to be one significant problem: physicians are not, as a rule, providing clear, understandable dictation, and are not furnishing it consistently within the institution's required 15-day period. Perhaps also the various facets of this apparently sizeable difficulty have been identified as the following: many physicians are not dictating within the required period, so the necessary procedure is not being followed; many physicians have complained about unavailable dictating equipment or dictating equipment that operates poorly or not at all, so there are equipment difficulties; there have been numerous complaints about ineffective sound-deadening in the dictation area, and dictating stations are cramped closely together; there are only two setups available to handle the taping of telephone dictation, and physicians complain that the lines are always tied up. Thus the total problem may be divided into several sub-problems, each of which may be addressed separately, at least at first: 1) the physicians' recording procedure; 2) the state of the dictation equipment; 3) the physical environment of the dictation area; and 4) the telephone dictation system. Once the problems have been separately addressed and tentative solutions developed, these sub-solutions may be combined and integrated into a solution to the total problem. Thus a single problem that may prove to be excessively unwieldy when tackled in the whole can often be approached as a series of more manageable sub-problems.

Challenge Everything

All of the information gathered to this point, especially the record of how a particular task is now being done, must be subjected to searching study. Nothing is to be taken for granted. At every step along the way, it is necessary to ask: What is actually being done? Where is it being done? How is it done? And always, for every step, it is necessary to ask: Why is it being done?

Every step should be examined and every detail should be challenged in an effort to:

- Eliminate activities whenever possible. Just because somethng is being done is no reason why it must be done. It is necessary to ask of each step: If this were not done at all, what would be the result?
- Combine steps whenever possible.
- Improve the manner of performing various steps.
- Change sequences of activities, locations of work stations, assignments of people involved, and other factors that might have a bearing on efficient task performance.

The process of challenging every detail lies at the heart of methods improvement. It is here that methods improvement, while appearing to many to be a logical scientific approach, must become a wide open, no-holds-barred creative process. It is here that participation and teamwork have far-reaching implications. The use of brainstorming and other creative idea-generating techniques; the importance of optimism, other "up" attitudes, and genuine belief in the necessity for improvement; the willingness to experiment, to innovate, to fail occasionally as part of the learning process and to try the untried; the knowledge of the tools and techniques of information gathering and analysis; the complete involvement of all parties who have a stake in the problem, regardless of their level in the organization; and a healthy, positive attitude toward the need for constructive change—all of these come together in challenging every detail of the problem and carrying the problem solvers toward the results of the next step.

Develop an Improved Method

Having thoroughly learned about the task and having uncovered both its weaknesses and strengths, it is possible to use the results of this analysis to develop a proposed new method. However, the process is not as simple as replacing the old method with the new method with no further preparation. Rather, it is necessary to:

- Thoroughly check the proposed method using flowcharts and other analytical techniques, subjecting the new method to the same kind of detailed examination that was applied to the present method, to provide reasonable assurance that the difficulties that led to the consideration of this task have been corrected.

- Since the effective application of the resulting new method will fall to the people who actually do the work day to day, analyze the potential impact of the proposed method in terms of human involvement. The best methods-engineered procedure ever to reach the department is bound for eventual failure if it includes elements that the worker—the critical human factor—considers demeaning or dissatisfying. When the "perfect" solution (perfect in a technical sense) is combined with the human element, it is sometimes necessary to retreat from technical perfection to accommodate the needs of employees. For example, productive efficiency in a large hospital's highly automated personnel department might suggest that one personnel assistant should sit at a video display terminal (VDT) for eight hours each day and put into the system all necessary activity. It is highly likely, however, that such a rigid assignment—with the person essentially chained to a chair, keyboard, and screen all day—will lead to the physical discomfort of backache and eyestrain and the intellectual numbness born of repetition and boredom, and lead to dissatisfaction that often results in reduced efficiency and diminished productivity. It is better to sacrifice some theoretical efficiency up front, perhaps by rearranging the work of this person and another so that both alternately divide their time between the necessary VDT activities and other nonterminal activities.
- If possible, make trial runs of experimental applications to test the proposed method. In this way it is also possible to test variations in methods to determine which might work better in practice or which might be more palatable to the employees who do the work.
- In general, the practicability of the proposed method should be assessed in the light of any constraints that may be present. It is one thing to idealize a method; it is another matter to make that method work in the face of constraints provided by limitations on cost, time, and quality considerations. There are usually limits on these factors—one can spend only so much, the task must be accomplished within a given length of time, and quality must ordinarily be maintained at present levels or perhaps even improved—and the workable solution must fall within these limits.

Implement and Follow Up

Action is a must. The best work method ever devised is useless as long as it remains solely on paper.

One should be prepared to accept a certain amount of necessary "tuning up" and "debugging." Steps that appear to work well on paper often require modification in practice. Also, conditions are constantly changing, and needs and circumstances present at the time of implementation may be different from those existing when the analysis was started. Rarely is a plan of any consequence implemented 100 percent as planned, so one must be ready to deal with implementation until all irregularities have been worked out.

Be aware of potential human relations problems and of the value of employee participation in methods improvement. Often the extent of participation that may have preceded implementation will have already determined the success or failure of a proposed new method.

Human problems encountered in the implementation of new work procedures are often the classic problems of resistance to change. To make additional but necessary mention of employee participation, there is usually an identifiable relationship between employee involvement ānd employee resistance to change: the more intimately involved employees are in determining the form and substance of a change, the more likely they are to accept that change and be less resistant. When implementing new methods or procedures or in general instituting any change, the supervisor has three available avenues of approach. The supervisor can:

1) *Tell the employees what to do.* This would perhaps at the time seem to be the simplest, most straightforward way of getting something done. However, simple telling, that is, giving direct orders only, more often than not creates resentment, unsettles the employees, and frequently breeds resistance. There will occasionally be some employees who simply have to be told, but these will probably be relatively few, so the direct-order approach should always be the last resort in attempting to get employees to do something new.

2) *Convince the employees of what must be done.* Not always is there the opportunity for true participation of employees in determining what a new method or process or task will be. Sometimes—as in instances when new or altered methods must be put in place in response to edicts from higher management or mandates from regulatory agencies—even the supervisor may have no voice in determining the direction of change. In such an instance, however, the supervisor (and the supervisor's boss) can make every effort to "sell" the concerned employees on the change and convince them to go along. All personnel involved at all organizational levels are more likely to comply with what is required if they know and understand *why* something must be done. At the least, each employee in the department deserves to know the why of every task.

3) *Involve employees in determining the form and substance of the change.*
This is of course the recommended route to take whenever possible. It is usually possible unless the particular change is one resulting from an edict or man-
date referred to earlier. Regarding methods improvement, employee involvement in determining new and revised methods is advisable for a number of
important reasons including:

- The employee who is thus involved will be thoroughly knowledgeable
  of the details of the new method as it is created.
- The involved employee will "own a piece" of the new method and will
  be more likely to accept that method.
- The employee is one of the most valuable sources, if not the single most
  valuable source, of information concerning how the task is now performed and how it might better be performed. The supervisor may have
  the superior perspective of departmental operations and may be able to
  stand back and observe that pieces do not fit together well and that a
  number of things need to be improved. However, the employees who
  perform these specific tasks day in and day out know best of all people
  the inner working details. This source of information should not be
  allowed to go untapped in methods improvement.

Close follow-up on implementation is essential, and for many tasks it must
be maintained for a considerable length of time. Time is necessary for new
habits to form and replace old habits, for new methods to dominate
employees' actions completely and negate any fond remembrances of "the
way we used to do it." Also, any newly installed method is immediately subject to unforeseen problems and creeping changes that can affect performance. Thus it is necessary to follow up a new method until it has taken its
place completely among the department's normal processes; even then this
method, as with all of a department's procedures, should be subject to
periodic audit of effectiveness and appropriateness.

TOOLS AND TECHNIQUES OF METHODS IMPROVEMENT

A number of analytical tools and techniques are available to a person pursuing methods improvement. Only a few such techniques will be introduced
in this chapter; these will be relatively easy to use and applicable to many
situations.

One of the most valuable tools available for examining an activity is the
flow process chart, used for tracking and recording the steps of an activity
and assessing the nature of each step. Flow process charts appear in many

forms but most make use of the five activity symbols shown in Figure 8-1. For proper analysis all work activity should be divided into at least these five basic categories:

1) An operation is any activity that advances the completion of the task. It is the actual performance of work, whether it be writing on a form, dialing a telephone, giving an injection, making a photocopy, tightening a bolt, or whatever.

Figure 8-1 Flow Process Chart Symbols

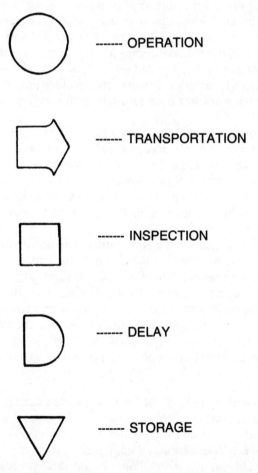

Source: Reprinted from Charles R. McConnell, *The Effective Health Care Supervisor* (Rockville, Md.: Aspen Systems Corp., 1982), p. 254.

2) A transportation represents any movement encountered in the process. It may be the movement of a patient from here to there, the delivery of a memo from an employee to the supervisor, the carrying of a record to the copy machine, or any other activity in which movement is the primary characteristic. Note that transportation involves only physical movement; except for the relocation of some person or thing from one place to another, nothing actually happens to advance the completion of the work—for instance, the chart that just arrived on person B's desk in Medical Records is just as incomplete as when it left person A's hands on the nursing floor.

3) An inspection is an activity in which the primary emphasis is verification of the results of prior operations. For instance, a housekeeping supervisor may periodically check areas that have been recently cleaned; an admitting supervisor may check an admission form to assure it is appropriately completed; a business office supervisor may assign an employee the task of verifying statements before they are sent out. Inspections, like transportations, do not advance the completion of work. Rather, they are used to determine whether necessary work has been properly performed.

4) A delay is an unplanned interruption in the flow of necessary steps. A pencil breaks and must be replaced; a typewriter jams and must be cleared; a beverage spills, necessitating cleanup and replacement; a waiting line is encountered at the central supply window; the person who must sign the hand-carried requisition is busy on the telephone—all of these are examples of delays that might be encountered in flow process analysis.

5) A storage is indicated when a step results in an anticipated interruption in the process, or it may represent the end of the process. More in-depth analysis than that presented here often calls for carefully distinguishing between temporary and permanent storage. For example, the completed bill just placed in the mailroom out-basket is in temporary storage; the process will be resumed after some period of time. However, although the complete medical record recently filed on the shelf may be retrieved sometime in the future, it is for all practical purposes in permanent storage.

Although the activity symbols of Figure 8-1 can be used in charting work activity in freehand fashion, they are ordinarily incorporated into prepared forms. A simplified version of a portion of a flow process chart form appears in Exhibit 8-1. If this form is used, it is necessary only to describe each activity, preferably in no more than two or three words; indicate the appropriate symbol for that activity; and, as one may wish, connect the symbols to indicate the sequential flow of activities.

Exhibit 8-1 Flow Process Chart (Form)

	SUMMARY			PROCEDURE CHARTED	

		PRESENT		PROPOSED		SAVINGS	
		NO	HRS	NO	HRS	NO	HRS
○	OPERATION						
⇨	TRANSPORT						
▪	INSPECTION						
D	DELAY						
▽	STORAGE						

PROCEDURE CHARTED

PERSON ☐ MATERIAL ☐

CHART BEGINS — CHART ENDS

CHARTED BY — DATE

DISTANCE TRAVELED   ☐ PRESENT   ☐ PROPOSED

#	STEPS IN PROCEDURE	OPERATIONS	DIST. IN FT.	TIME IN HRS.	REMARKS
1		○⇨▪D▽			
2		○⇨▪D▽			
3		○⇨▪D▽			
4		○⇨▪D▽			
5		○⇨▪D▽			
6		○⇨▪D▽			
7		○⇨▪D▽			
8		○⇨▪D▽			
9		○⇨▪D▽			
10		○⇨▪D▽			
11		○⇨▪D▽			
12		○⇨▪D▽			
13		○⇨▪D▽			
14		○⇨▪D▽			
15		○⇨▪D▽			
16		○⇨▪D▽			
17		○⇨▪D▽			
18		○⇨▪D▽			
19		○⇨▪D▽			

APPROVED BY   TOTALS   PAGE OF PAGES

Source: Reprinted from Charles R. McConnell, The Effective Health Care Supervisor (Rockville, Md.: Aspen Systems Corp., 1982), p. 255.

An important indicator of the proper use of the flow process chart is embodied in the need for the user to note whether the chart follows the activities of a person or the flow of material. This decision must be made before beginning the analysis. For example, if a clerk who is preparing and then processing a three-part form is observed, a point may soon be reached in the activity at which the form is taken apart and proceeds to flow in three directions while the clerk either remains working with one part of the form or may go off in a fourth and completely different direction. It is thus necessary for the user to make an early decision on the focus of the analysis (for example, either "purchase requisition" or "purchasing clerk" and stay with it throughout.

There is space on the chart for summary of total numbers of work activities and total distances traveled in transportation steps, which is convenient for comparing possible changes with present methods.

Another simple but helpful tool is the flow diagram, a sample of which appears in Figure 8-2. A flow diagram is a layout drawing drawn to approx-

Figure 8-2 Flow Diagram Showing X-Ray Technician Travel

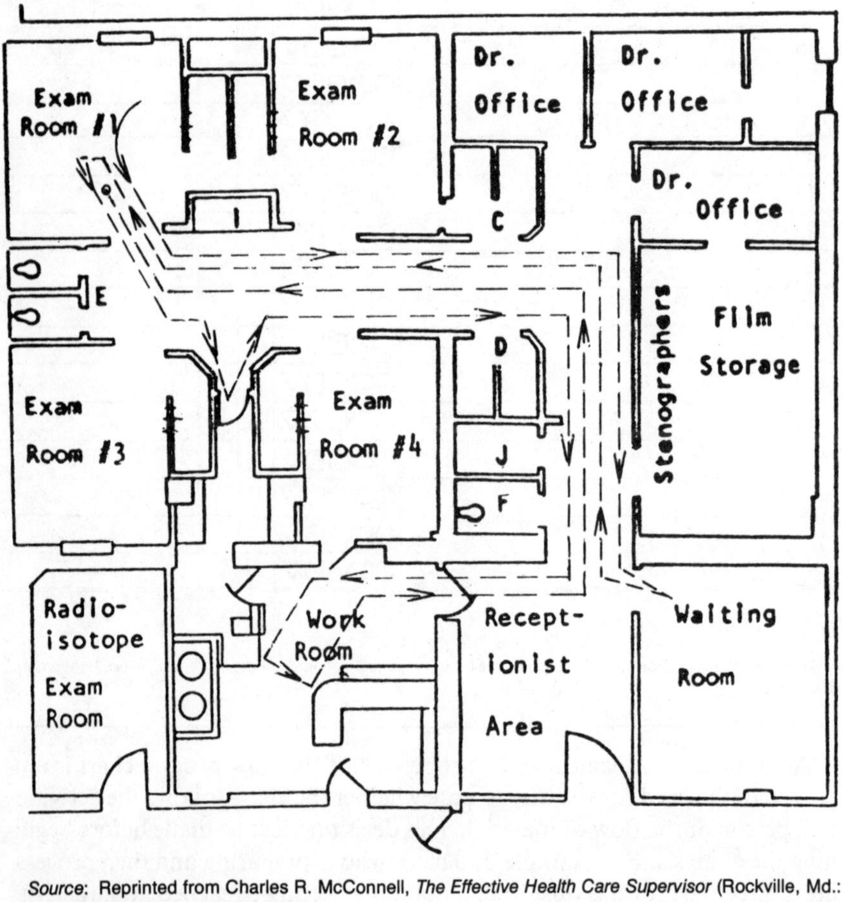

Source: Reprinted from Charles R. McConnell, *The Effective Health Care Supervisor* (Rockville, Md.: Aspen Systems Corp., 1982), p. 257.

imate scale, on which lines are placed to indicate paths of personnel movement or material flow. This diagram can be especially helpful in determining how to rearrange equipment, furnishings, and work stations for improved effectiveness. This technique may be used to assess the approximate amount of movement required by a particular layout, and any potential new layout may thus be tested on paper to determine whether it represents an improvement.

Numerous additional techniques are available for analyzing work activities. Some of these techniques are:

- *The Operation Process Chart.* Whereas a flow process chart captures an entire sequence of all operations, transportations, inspections, delays, and storages occurring during a process or activity, an operation process chart typically focuses only on operations (the circular symbol) and inspections (the square symbol). It is used most conveniently to examine all the separate small activities or suboperations that may occur within a larger task. For example, "Take chest x-ray" may appear as a single operation on a flow process chart covering the activities of an x-ray technician; however, if one wished to examine "Take chest x-ray" in detail one might focus on this activity alone and create an operation process chart that breaks it into a number of smaller work activities (operations) and verification steps (inspections).

- *Multiple Activity Flow Process Chart.* This tool would be most useful if one wished to examine, for example, a several-part form that is processed over a period of days. Utilizing the standard charting symbols, this chart would perhaps display the multiple parts of the subject form in a vertical column at the left and a time scale of perhaps several days of the week across the horizontal dimension. Using this technique one can illustrate, usually on a single sheet of paper, what happens to each part of the multi-part form on each day in the processing cycle.

- *Multiple Activity Chart.* Formerly referred to as a man-and-machine chart, this chart is used to trace the activities of an employee working in conjunction with one or more pieces of equipment. The heart of this chart is a vertical time scale calibrated in either minutes or decimal parts of an hour. Parallel with this time scale the activities of the worker are indicated and the utilization of the equipment is indicated. This technique makes it possible to identify those times when workers or equipment are waiting or being productively applied, and thus makes it possible to consider rearrangements of activity that may reduce idle (nonproductive) time for worker, equipment, or both.

- *Gang Process Chart.* This flow process chart is applied to the analysis of the activities of a crew of two or more persons who must work together to accomplish a given task. The steps taken by each member of the crew are charted in a time-scale relationship to each other; that is, what worker A is doing at any particular time appears directly beside the activity that worker B is performing at the same time.

As was the case with the discussion of the establishment of productivity standards (Chapter 6), this brief overview of methods improvement barely scratches the surface of management engineering technology. For the supervisor who may wish to pursue methods analysis in more detail, perhaps to the extent of being able to collaborate with management engineers in methods improvement projects or independently pursue such projects within the department, helpful published references are available. Three of the best such references, also cited in connection with the discussion on measuring and monitoring productivity, are:

- Ralph M. Barnes, *Motion and Time Study*, 7th ed. (New York: Wiley, 1980).
- H.B. Maynard, ed. *Industrial Engineering Handbook*, 3rd ed. (New York: McGraw-Hill, 1971).
- Harold E. Smalley, *Hospital Management Engineering: A Guide to Improvement of Hospital Management Systems* (Englewood Cliffs, N.J.: Prentice-Hall, 1982).

EXAMPLE: THE INFORMATION REQUEST

Exhibit 8-2 is a flow process chart of 17 steps illustrating the processing of a single information request in a medical record department. The activity begins when a request for information is pulled from the incoming mail; it ends when the fulfilled request is filed, that is, entered into storage, in the clerk's desk or file cabinet. The nature of the intervening steps should be evident from their brief descriptions.

With the complete task of answering an information request recorded on a flow process chart, one can begin to question the individual steps involved to determine whether there is room for improvement. For instance, observation has revealed that considerable travel is involved in what appears to be a small task—about 100 feet of walking. This should raise questions as to whether any furniture or nonpermanent fixtures could be relocated to reduce personnel travel.

The delay recorded on line 8, waiting for the copy machine to warm up, should raise questions. The delay may be legitimate—there are some copy

Exhibit 8-2 Flow Process Chart: Information Request (Single)

	SUMMARY				PROCEDURE CHARTED
		PRESENT NO HRS	PROPOSED NO HRS	SAVINGS NO HRS	*INFORMATION REQUEST (SINGLE)*

		PRESENT		PROPOSED		SAVINGS	
		NO	HRS	NO	HRS	NO	HRS
○	OPERATION	10					
⇨	TRANSPORT	3					
□	INSPECTION	1					
D	DELAY	1					
▽	STORAGE	2					

PERSON □ MATERIAL ☑

CHART BEGINS *GET REQUEST* CHART ENDS *FILE*

CHARTED BY *CRM* DATE *3/9/81*

DISTANCE TRAVELED *100' (FOR 1)* ☑ PRESENT   □ PROPOSED

	STEPS IN PROCEDURE	OPER.	TRANS	INSP.	DELAY	STORE	DIST. IN FT.	TIME IN HRS.	REMARKS
1	*GET, OPEN, & READ*	⊗	⇨	□	D	▽			
2	*VERIFY AUTHORIZATION*	○	⇨	☒	D	▽			
3	*GET CHART*	⊗	⇨	□	D	▽	15		
4	*CHART TO DESK*	○	⇨	□	D	▽	15		
5	*LOCATE & REMOVE PAGES*	⊗	⇨	□	D	▽			
6	*TO COPIER*	○	⇨	□	D	▽	20		
7	*START COPIER*	⊗	⇨	□	D	▽			
8	*WAIT FOR WARM-UP*	○	⇨	□	☒	▽			
9	*MAKE COPIES*	⊗	⇨	□	D	▽			
10	*RETURN TO DESK*	○	⇨	□	D	▽	20		
11	*RE-ASSEMBLE CHART*	⊗	⇨	□	D	▽			
12	*RE-FILE CHART*	○	⇨	□	D	▽	30		
13	*TYPE BILL & ENVELOPE*	⊗	⇨	□	D	▽			
14	*ASSEMBLE TO MAIL*	⊗	⇨	□	D	▽			
15	*INTO OUTGOING MAIL*	○	⇨	□	D	▽			
16	*ENTER IN LOG*	⊗	⇨	□	D	▽			
17	*FILE REQUEST*	○	⇨	□	D	▽			
18		○	⇨	□	D	▽			
19		○	⇨	□	D	▽			

APPROVED BY   TOTALS   PAGE   OF   PAGES

Source: Reprinted from Charles R. McConnell, The Effective Health Care Supervisor (Rockville, Md.: Aspen Systems Corp., 1982), p. 259.

machines that should be shut down between infrequent uses—but one will never discover this without probing to determine *why*.

It is also reasonable to consider whether certain steps could be eliminated or combined. For instance, is it possible to obtain the chart as in step 3, then go directly to the copy machine and perform the next several activities there and thus eliminate a pair of transportations? Or if the copy machine warmup should indeed be required, would it be productive for the employee to turn the machine on before getting the chart so the machine can be used without delay when needed?

Other pertinent questions should form as the chart is studied. However, the most important question relative to this example has not yet been raised: How many information requests are involved? If requests arrive at the clerk's in-basket in batches, several additional questions become important:

- Can these requests be processed in batches, doing each step for several requests at a time?
- Can all necessary charts be obtained at once?
- Would it be practical to save all bill preparation for one time of day?
- Should all filing be done at the end of the day?
- Should physical changes be considered, such as moving a desk, to reduce transportation distances?

In the actual situation from which this example was taken, mail arrived in the medical record department once in the morning and once in the afternoon. The clerk was in the habit of running information requests twice a day, usually within an hour or so of the arrival of mail, whether the batch consisted of a single request or several requests. A few simple changes in procedure were indicated:

- The copy machine was turned on at the beginning of the day and left on (investigation showed this to be the manufacturer's recommendation). It was decided to run the requests in batches, with little change in the steps indicated (trial runs involving a clerk doing several steps at the copy machine produced a situation that was awkward and thus counterproductive).
- An ideal batch size of 10 to 12 requests was established, thus providing that no request went unanswered longer than two days (the decision was to run 10 to 12 at once or a maximum of two days' requests, whichever accumulated first).
- A simple change in layout—turning the clerk's desk around and moving it about eight feet—reduced total travel from 100 feet to 70 feet (a flow chart of the resulting activity appears as Exhibit 8-3).

The amount of effort put into such an analysis will depend largely on the total workload involved. In the situation just described, for example, if information requests amounted only to one or two a day, as might be the case in a very small hospital, little can be gained by shaving a minute or so from

Exhibit 8-3 Flow Process Chart: Information Request (Batch)

	SUMMARY	PRESENT NO	PRESENT HRS	PROPOSED NO	PROPOSED HRS	SAVINGS NO	SAVINGS HRS	PROCEDURE CHARTED
○	OPERATION	9						*INFORMATION REQUEST (BATCH)*
⟶	TRANSPORT	3						PERSON ☐ MATERIAL ☑
☐	INSPECTION	1						CHART BEGINS *GET REQUESTS* CHART ENDS *FILE*
D	DELAY	0						CHARTED BY *CRM* DATE *3/9/81*
▽	STORAGE	2						

DISTANCE TRAVELED *70' (FOR 10-12)* ☐ PRESENT   ☑ PROPOSED

	STEPS IN PROCEDURE	OPER.	TRANS.	INSP.	DELAY	STORE.	DIST. IN FT.	TIME IN HRS.	REMARKS
1	*GET, OPEN, READ, & SORT BY #*	●	○	☐	D	▽			*MAX. 10-12/BATCH*
2	*VERIFY AUTHORIZATIONS*	○	○	☑	D	▽			
3	*GET CHARTS*	●	○	☐	D	▽	10		
4	*CHARTS TO DESK*	○	●	☐	D	▽	10		
5	*LOCATE & REMOVE PAGES*	●	○	☐	D	▽			
6	*TO COPIER*	○	●	☐	D	▽	15		
7	*MAKE COPIES*	●	○	☐	D	▽			
8	*RETURN TO DESK*	○	●	☐	D	▽	15		
9	*RE-ASSEMBLE CHARTS*	●	○	☐	D	▽			
10	*RE-FILE CHARTS*	●	○	☐	D	▽	20		
11	*TYPE BILLS & ENVELOPES*	●	○	☐	D	▽			
12	*ASSEMBLE TO MAIL*	●	○	☐	D	▽			
13	*INTO OUTGOING MAIL*	○	○	☐	D	▼			
14	*ENTER IN LOG*	●	○	☐	D	▽			
15	*FILE REQUESTS*	○	○	☐	D	▼			
16		○	○	☐	D	▽			
17		○	○	☐	D	▽			
18		○	○	☐	D	▽			
19		○	○	☐	D	▽			

APPROVED BY   TOTALS   PAGE   OF   PAGES

Source: Reprinted from Charles R. McConnell, *The Effective Health Care Supervisor* (Rockville, Md.: Aspen Systems Corp., 1982), p. 262.

each repetition of the task. The time of the supervisor or other work analyst is as valuable as the time of the employee, and hours of effort can be wasted to produce obviously minuscule returns. Under conditions of high volume, however, there may be significant gains to be made through a few hours' effort. If, for instance, the institution is of sufficient size that processing such requests requires one or more full-time persons, analysis could help decide whether one person could or could not do the job alone. As early as possible in the methods improvement process, one should assess the potential savings in time and resources. Always, one's best efforts should be directed toward improvements that show the greatest potential for savings in time or other resources.

AN ORGANIZED APPROACH TO METHODS IMPROVEMENT

A formal, institution-wide methods improvement program should ordinarily consist of three phases: philosophy, education, and application.

Philosophy

The belief in continuous methods improvement effort and in the need for a formal methods improvement program should exist at the top of the organization. For a program to be successful over the long run, top management should be active and visible. Regardless of where the idea begins, top management must be seen by all employees of the organization as 100 percent behind an organized effort to maintain constant cost containment pressure through continuous, positive questioning of work methods. This commitment must be reflected in a shared belief that there are few activities that cannot be improved.

The dissemination of the methods improvement philosophy throughout the organization may require much promotional effort. Promoting the benefits of continuous oversight of work methods will necessarily be a selling job that is never truly complete, although once a program is under way and some positive results have been generated these results will in turn help to sell the philosophy. The guiding philosophy of a methods improvement program must proceed downward from administration through every member of the management organization and to every employee in the work force. Through meetings large and small and through printed matter of various forms everyone in the organization should receive and be encouraged to retain the basic message: Cost containment is here to stay, and continuing attention to making each hour of human labor and each dollar's worth of material input go farther and do better and produce better quality results is one of the important ways we can all help to keep the institution solvent and thus continue to serve our patients and protect our jobs.

Education

Some weeks after the initial institution-wide introduction of the methods improvement philosophy, the process of educating people in the tools and techniques of methods improvement should begin. Taking a form similar to that described in the example in Chapter 7 concerning the multi-hospital training program in methods improvement might bring supervisors and managers together with management engineering and industrial engineering professionals and begin to acquaint them with the ways and means of work analysis. Should this education be pursued in the manner described in the example cited, that is, with supervisors bringing actual problems from the job into the classroom, the education process would also provide some initial pilot projects that could carry into the application phase of methods improvement.

During the education phase, and after a number of supervisors and managers have been partially oriented to a working knowledge of methods improvement tools and techniques, it would be helpful to begin bringing non-supervisory employees—especially those with skills likely to be called upon on future projects—into the education process.

Application

Ideally the ongoing application of a methods improvement program should be pursued under the guidance and oversight of either an administrative steering committee or a methods improvement coordinator who is a member of administration (preferably) or a management engineer or industrial engineer (desirably) or both (ideally). In addition to providing active assistance and coordinating necessary skills and resources, the primary role of the steering committee or coordinator is to keep methods improvement projects moving. Methods improvement will necessarily not always be particularly high on the average supervisor's list of priorities; there is usually more than enough to be done without bothering with such. Thus in constantly monitoring the program, the steering committee or coordinator serves as a constant reminder that periodic activity is required to keep methods improvement alive, and also makes the entire process easier for supervisors involved in active projects.

As suggested earlier, some of the first projects undertaken within a methods improvement program could be those that emerge as pilot projects pursued originally within the context of a methods improvement educational program. When pursuing such projects early in the undertaking, it is advisable to pursue initially those projects that carry the greatest potential returns or that are most easily concluded. Although this may seem like "skimming the cream" or going after just "the easy stuff," there is a distinct advantage in doing so: some early visible successes often serve as a much needed boost to provide momentum to the entire program.

Individual project teams may take two forms: the ad hoc group assembled for a single project, or the ongoing group formed to deal with a particular department or specific function.

The ideal ad hoc project team might consist of:

- the person responsible for the performance of the job (the supervisor);
- the assistant to the person responsible for the job, if there is one;
- one or two of the persons who regularly do the job day to day;
- one expert from outside the department who is knowledgeable in the most prominent technical specialty related to the job (for example, an accountant to deal with aspects of a billing problem, a materials management specialist to deal with a transportation problem, a personnel specialist to deal with personnel policy issues).

For an ongoing project team, one that might deal with a series of projects relating to a particular department or a specific function within a department, the ideal team might consist of:

- the department head or assistant department head;
- a representative of administration;
- a representative of the organization's finance division;
- a management engineer, industrial engineer, or systems analyst;
- one or more expert positions, to be filled by persons from technical specialties involved in particular projects;
- at least one nonsupervisory employee of the department.

If much of the foregoing appears idealistic—and with the history of such undertakings, where in many organizations much has been started but most has died or gradually dwindled to nothing, these aims may seem idealistic—there is nevertheless the opportunity for the individual supervisor to pursue methods improvement strictly within the confines of his or her own department. There are some projects that can never be undertaken or successfully completed without interdepartmental cooperation. However, such projects aside, there exist within each department countless ways in which a conscientious supervisor and a few positively motivated employees can improve work methods and contain costs. In the average operating department of any health care institution a great deal of improvement can be accomplished if the supervisor recognizes the possibilities for improvement and provides the example of leadership required to bring the employees into the improvement process.

THE METHODS-MINDED ATTITUDE

The methods-minded attitude referred to earlier has its foundation in each employee's belief that improvement is always possible, and that, if left alone for prolonged periods, work activities will experience creeping changes that are usually not for the better. Methods mindedness will often be reflected in the person who develops efficient work habits and always approaches a task so as to achieve satisfactory results with minimum effort. Methods mindedness, then, might seem to be a talent. Rather, however, it is a habit, or, more appropriately, a collection of habits. As a habit, methods mindedness can be learned. The supervisor's attitude toward methods improvement will be most important in encouraging the employees to become methods minded as well. The supervisor need not plunge into methods improvement in a full-scale manner; rather, attention should be limited to one or two troublesome tasks at a time, or to one activity or process that seems to hold room for improvement. Even if only one such project is open at a time, with the supervisor and others working on it as time allows or can be made, noticeable progress is bound to accrue, and as a result the interest of some of the employees will be stimulated. Employees who actually do the work can see much that is hidden from the supervisor regarding working procedural details.

Part IV

People: Making Best Use of the Ultimate Resource

Chapter 9

Staffing and Scheduling

A little neglect may breed great mischief.

Benjamin Franklin

Chapter Objectives

- Outline the requirements of effective staffing and illustrate the application of a departmental staffing standard.
- Introduce the concept of variable staffing and illustrate its application.
- Recommend ways and means of adjusting for conditions of overstaffing and understaffing.
- Describe the basic scheduling environments and highlight the policies that should exist in support of effective scheduling.
- Introduce and illustrate cyclical scheduling.
- Survey the advantages and disadvantages of relying on the use of part-time employees.
- Explore the concept of "flextime" and other nonconventional work schedules.

SIDES OF THE SAME COIN

In practiced, the terms *staffing* and *scheduling* are often used together to refer to a general process, and not infrequently they are used separately to mean essentially the same thing. However, although they are as firmly related to each other as two sides of the same coin, there are nevertheless differences between staffing and scheduling that at times mark them as separate processes. These differences are highlighted in the following comparisons:

- Staffing is determining how many people of what specific skills are needed and when they are needed, and assuring their availability.
- Scheduling is bringing human resources together in a time relationship with the work to be done. Scheduling involves determining who (specifically by name and skill) will do what work and when (specifically by designated time period).

In viewing the supervisor's role in terms of basic management functions, staffing is essentially part of organizing, that is, establishing the framework within which the work is to be done and determining who will do what. On the other hand, scheduling, although it also deals with who will do what plus the added dimension of when, is an integral part of the basic management function of planning. Indeed, scheduling is one of the two most refined forms of planning (the other is budgeting) that a supervisor will encounter in operating a department. A personnel schedule is no more or less than a short-term plan expressed as people arranged relative to days or shifts or other blocks of time.

The supervisor's role in making staffing decisions and becoming involved in scheduling will necessarily vary according to the policies and practices of the institution. Depending on institution policies, organization structure, and the individual department or function involved, the supervisor can be involved minimally or totally immersed in the processes.

Effective staffing and scheduling hold important cost-related implications for today's health care supervisor. Statistics published in mid-1984 revealed that 53.1 percent of total hospital expense nationwide went for wages and salaries and another 8.1 percent went for employee benefits related to those wages and salaries; thus current information shows that more than 61 percent of every dollar spent by every hospital goes for staff.[1] Therefore, to control departmental staffing levels and to schedule employees efficiently for maximum effect means controlling 60 percent or more of the budget. This chapter will examine the major aspects of staffing and scheduling as related to the role of the supervisor.

STAFFING

Although staffing is primarily the consideration of how many people of what skills may be required, the process must be tempered throughout by scheduling considerations.

Reasonably accurate staffing requires the use of a staffing standard, essentially a productivity standard that includes adjustments for personal time, fatigue and delay time, target utilization, and the like. (Refer to Chapter 6, Measuring and Monitoring Productivity.)

Consider the productivity standard for the hypothetical medical record department described in Chapter 6:

22.8 hours/calendar day + 1.746 hours/discharge.

It is necessary to combine such a standard with reliable knowledge of work activity to determine the department's required staffing.

Example: Application of a Staffing Standard

If the year-round average volume in the sample medical record department is 671 discharges per four-week period, one can determine the staffing required to meet that projected volume. In abbreviated, simplified fashion, one would proceed as follows:

- The 671 discharges per four-week period translate into 8,723 discharges per year.
- One full-time equivalent (FTE) employee works 40 hours per week or 2,080 hours per year.
- So: $$\frac{(22.8 \text{ hrs} \times 365 \text{ days}) + (1.746 \text{ hrs} \times 8,723 \text{ discharges})}{2,080 \text{ hrs}}$$

$$\frac{8,322 + 15,230}{2,080} = \frac{23,552}{2,080} = 11.3 \text{ FTE}.$$

Thus 11.3 FTEs actively at work should be required to support the average volume of 671 discharges per four-week period (or an average of 727 discharges per month, since work-volume statistics may be forecast or maintained by month rather than by four-week period).

The foregoing refers only to a requirement for 11.3 FTEs actually working. However, since a significant amount of time not worked is nevertheless paid for, it becomes necessary to compensate for this difference in determining total staffing. To account for the effects of time-paid-not-worked—primarily vacations, holidays, and sick time (VHS factor)—in this particular medical record department it is known that:

- Based on employees' work status and length of service, four people receive four weeks of vacation (20 days) per year, three employees receive three weeks (15 days) per year, and the balance of the employees receive two weeks vacation (10 days) per year. Assume that all staff members in toto earn 168 vacation days in a year.
- All employees of the institution receive 10 paid holidays per year, so on the average this department accounts for 113 paid holidays per year (10 days × 11.3 FTEs, calculated on the assumption that customary practices apply and part-time employees receive holidays and certain other benefits in proportion to their work schedules).
- Average sick time usage is 4.7 days per employee per year, so the department may be expected to consume an average of 53 paid sick days per year.

Together the foregoing items amount to a probable average 334 days per year that the department will pay for employees who are legitimately absent from work. In addition, this also means that 334 days worth of work needs to be covered by employees who *are* present. Time-paid-not-worked is a built-in part of the employment relationship and must be accounted for in determining required staff; a given level of employee presence actually on the job is required to accomplish the work, but a somewhat greater employee presence must be bought and paid for to assure the required level of staff at work.

To continue the example: 334 full work days equal 2,672 hours. Then:

$$\frac{2,672}{2,080} = 1.3 \text{ FTE}.$$

On the average, to maintain an FTE of 11.3, the example above requires 12.6 FTEs of paid staff to compensate for time-paid-not-worked. Or, expressed in another way:

$$\frac{12.6}{12.6 - 1.3} = \frac{12.6}{11.3} = 1.115 \text{ VHS factor}.$$

Another 11.5 percent must be added to required staff to compensate for vacations, holidays, and sick time.

A VHS factor can be determined for any individual department much as in the preceding paragraphs; however, this factor may already exist as a flat percentage applied to all departments throughout the institution. Although the latter is often the case, it often pays to examine the time-paid-not-worked situation within a particular department and adopt a department-specific VHS factor when deemed necessary. As a general rule, however, differences in the VHS factor may be critical only in the case of a very "young" department (turnover is high and vacation entitlement is uniformly low) or in a very old department (turnover is minimal and vacation entitlement is considerably higher than the institution's average).

Again consider the example, in which the VHS factor of 11.5 percent stems in part from the employees who earn an average three weeks' vacation. If all of these medical record employees averaged only two weeks vacation, the department's VHS factor would be 9.7 percent; if all of them averaged four weeks vacation, the department's VHS factor would be 13.2 percent. Thus it may at times be advisable to determine a VHS factor for an individual department. Also, it may be advisable to consider another influence in determining VHS for a particular department. The determination just reviewed proceeds on the assumption that employees who are absent must be replaced; however, if people are not replaced when absent (as might be the case for reasonable absences experienced in a personnel department, accounting department, or other support activity), considerably less VHS coverage may need to be built into the standard.

In general, the most directly applicable kind of staffing standard available is simply a productivity standard that has been adjusted to include an allowance for time-paid-not-worked.

Variable Staffing

Obviously, appropriately controlled personnel costs can contribute to the economic viability of the institution. Certainly the importance of economic viability has been increasing. Emerging providers such as preferred provider organizations (PPOs) and health maintenance organizations (HMOs), and even capital markets (sources of loans) are drawn toward institutions that can demonstrate the most reasonable personnel costs. An institution that has more flexibility in adjusting staffing levels to match real needs is thus more able to adapt to the changing health care environment and to a sometimes drastically fluctuating patient census. Variable or adjustable staffing provides such flexibility in managing costs.

Where it appears to be appropriate, one can apply variable staffing in conjunction with knowledge of expected variations in workload. Consider Table 9-1, an illustration of simplified variable staffing for the hypothetical medical record department of the continuing example. Assume that the institution is subject to the variable workload indicated, as might be the case in a facili-

Table 9-1 Variable Staffing Illustration

Four-Week Period Ending	Projected Activity (Discharges)	Required Staff	
		FTE Worked	FTE Paid
1/26/85	470	9.1	10.1
2/23/85	475	9.2	10.3
3/23/85	595	10.5	11.7
4/20/85	650	11.1	12.4
5/18/85	790	12.6	14.0
6/15/85	870	13.5	15.1
7/13/85	875	13.5	15.1
8/10/85	870	13.5	15.1
9/7/85	860	13.4	14.9
10/5/85	740	12.1	13.5
11/2/85	525	9.7	10.8
11/30/85	485	9.3	10.4
12/28/85	470	9.1	10.1

ty located in a resort community, and further assume that a number of years' experience permits the prediction of the volume levels identified as projected activity.

In considering staffing for this department, one should be interested in both worked staff (those who must be on hand) and paid staff (the required work staff plus a reasonable allowance for time-paid-not-worked). Note that required paid staff ranges from a low of 10.1 FTEs in December and January to a high of 15.1 during the period including June, July, and August. In addition, worked staff ranges from a low of 9.1 FTEs to a high of 13.5 FTEs. Average staffing, readily determined, is 11.3 worked FTEs or 12.6 paid FTEs.

Much of the managerial reasoning encountered before the advent of serious cost containment automatically favored staffing for maximum or near-maximum conditions. The rationale generally offered was on the order of: "We *must* be able to handle the maximum expected workload at any time." However, staffing the department at 13.5 worked FTEs and 15.1 paid FTEs would create significant imbalance. For 4 periods of the year staffing would be accurate; for 2 additional periods it would be about 7 to 12 percent over desired levels, still within tolerable limits. However, for 7 of 13 periods staffing levels would be from 22 to 48 percent above that required to do the necessary work. The department would be overstaffed to some extent, much of the time intolerably so, for nearly 70 percent of the year.

One alternative to staffing for maximum conditions might be to staff for supposed average conditions and then take other steps to compensate for conditions above or below average as they occur. If the department were to staff year round for average conditions (11.3 percent FTE), this would leave the department from 7 to 20 percent understaffed for nearly half a year (from late April or early May to sometime in September) and 2 to 24 percent overstaffed for the balance of the year. This is closer to fiscal practicality than staffing all year for maximum conditions, but it is still poor because of the existence of intolerable understaffing for lengthy periods and wasted resources during periods of overstaffing.

However, staffing for average conditions, or at least for some level below peak activity, is an appropriate start. With core staffing set at 11.3 worked FTEs and 12.6 paid FTEs, the supervisor of the department might:

For the half year of understaffing:

- Use temporary employees, adding either full-time or part-time temporary employees to the institution's payroll (for periods of six months or less), or using temporary help from personnel agencies.
- Expand the hours of existing part-time employees for the period of need.
- Fill short-term needs with the judicious use of overtime (refer to Chapter 10, Keeping Overtime under Control).
- Utilize per diem or optional employees from a carefully developed list of call-ins who agree to work occasional days to fill short-term staffing needs.
- Rearrange vacation policies so employees are encouraged to take vacation during times of nonpeak workload. This could involve, for instance, limiting the length of vacations that can be taken during periods of high activity.

For the half year of overstaffing:

- Rely on rearranged vacation policies to encourage more vacation during periods of nonpeak activity. Under such policies paid FTEs would remain elevated but the department would be removing most of its vacation obligation during periods when people could be spared most, so worked FTEs would be reduced.
- Reduce the hours of part-time staff as possible.
- Consider reducing some staff from full-time to part-time as these persons might be willing (but do so with assurance to employees that pension eligibility and other key benefits would not be affected).
- Consider the use of the credit day. Under the credit day concept, full-time employees can voluntarily take an occasional day off with permission during periods of low activity. No pay is received for a day not worked, but the employee is given credit for benefits as though the time

were worked. This approach builds in nominal cost for the continuation of full benefits, but it saves the larger cost of direct wages.

- Consistent with the institution's policy, allow informal leave, that is, additional unpaid time off, for employees who wish to take extended vacation trips during slack periods or who simply wish to take more time off. As long as it is consistently made available to all employees affected by workload variations, this approach will draw occasional interest, perhaps just enough to help a department over a potentially expensive slack period.
- Have clear, concise defendable policies in writing to support all of the foregoing suggested actions, policies that tie all such adjustment activities to the varying level of the workload.

Constant Attention Required

If the workload of the department remains reasonably steady throughout the year, the supervisor need not spend much time worrying about staffing. Once the required core staffing has been established and people have been secured for all positions, it may be necessary only occasionally to apply some of the simpler techniques for handling brief periods of understaffing, such as using temporary employees or increasing the hours of part-time workers, to compensate for employee sick time, medical leave, military leave, and such. However, if the department's workload is variable, the supervisor must apply constant attention to maintaining staffing levels as closely as possible to the actual workload.

Since newer approaches to health care reimbursement, and probably most future reimbursement approaches, are directly tied to volume of service, it will be necessary for the supervisor to maintain staffing as closely as possible to actual activity levels to keep personnel costs in a favorable relationship with revenue. To succeed in doing so, the supervisor must:

- Have a staffing standard that reasonably relates required staff to the department's basic unit of output (such as the example medical record department standard of 22.8 hours/calendar day plus 1.746 hours/discharge, or perhaps the standard for a particular nursing unit of 4.8 nursing hours/patient day).
- Know the department's level of activity and be able to reasonably predict major fluctuations in that level.
- Apply a thorough, consistent, and responsive approach to scheduling available people to work at the times they are needed.

SCHEDULING

Although often deceptively simple in concept, scheduling can be frustrating in practice because of the combined effects of:

- the institution's policies;
- collective bargaining agreements;
- labor laws;
- fringe benefit costs;
- personnel limitations, both in numbers of people and in specialities;
- employees' desires and preferences.

Whoever is doing the scheduling, whether supervisor or scheduling specialist, is always constrained by the foregoing limitations. In addition, all scheduling techniques are subject to two basic but severe shortcomings:

1. They cannot create personnel if such do not exist or are not available.
2. They cannot make people willingly work schedules that are undesirable or unacceptable to them.

Scheduling Environments

There are three basic scheduling environments. Based on the work patterns for which scheduling must be accomplished, these three environments are discussed in order of the scheduling difficulties they present.

1) *Traditional work week.* This is the basic Monday through Friday, 35- to 40-hour work week. The employees of the department are generally all on hand for the same time period. In health care institutions a number of supporting business activities are conducted within the framework of the traditional work week, including, for example, the accounting department, the personnel department, the administrative offices, and public relations. Generally there is little need for coverage beyond the normal work week, and usually there is no immediate relationship between staffing and fluctuations in units of service.

In the case of a function subject to the traditional work week, more often than not the schedule is simply the department's staffing pattern. Ordinarily all of the department's employees are in place during the same time periods each week—although starting and stopping times may differ slightly for some people—and work can largely be leveled, that is, much of the work can be adjusted to coincide with the presence of staff.

2) *Extended work week*. In the extended work week scheduling environment the basic five-day week must be covered and so must some part of weekends or some portion of evenings and perhaps nights. This is something less than seven-day, 24-hour coverage, but it includes known periods beyond the traditional work week during which coverage must be in place.

One example of the extended work week might be found in a medical record department that is open for four hours each evening and eight hours on Saturday. Another example might be a food service department that is open seven days each week but is regularly closed between 7:00 PM and 5:00 AM. Generally, this environment includes any department that is open for some part of the evening or night shift and weekends but covers times when no workers are present with people on call.

Under the extended work week, the person doing the scheduling is faced with some, although not all, of the problems encountered by schedulers working in the environment discussed next.

3) *Complete scheduled coverage*. Complete scheduled coverage applies to departments or functions in which some level of scheduled coverage is required 24 hours a day, seven days a week. This applies to all nursing units and it often applies to a number of clincial support departments. Depending on the institution's size and level of activity during so-called off hours, complete scheduled coverage may or may not be called for. For example, in a large metropolitan medical center the radiology department and the clinical laboratory will undoubtedly be staffed 24 hours a day, seven days a week (although staffing will be less at some times than others), but in a small rurual hospital these functions may not be staffed at all during off hours but will be covered as needed by people who are on call.

Scheduling Policies for Complete Coverage

1) *Weekends*. The policy concerning the frequency with which rotating personnel will work weekends probably has the greatest impact on scheduling practices of all policies related to scheduling. A policy of every third weekend off (two out of three weekends worked) enhances effective scheduling. However, the practice of scheduling to grant every other weekend off has been expanding for a number of years. A disporportionately large amount of weekend work has long been a factor making for dissatisfaction for many rotating health care workers, so many organizations, both through meeting collective bargaining demands and through taking similar action without union prodding, have aimed at the practice of granting every other weekend off. This creates some scheduling difficulties; there is no way that staff can be effectively scheduled under the every-other-weekend-off scheme unless the institution has a number of part-time employees equal to the number

of full-time employees on staff. Although every third weekend off readily facilitates the scheduling of rotating employees, it may be necessary to adopt or maintain an every-other-weekend-off policy for reasons of employee relations. Regardless of the weekend policy adopted, however, this policy should be consistently applied to all rotating employees.

2) *Part-time employees.* The policy for part-time staff concerning the number of weekends worked and other scheduling requirements should be the same as that applied to full-time staff. That is, if a full-time employee is expected to work all or part of every second weekend, a part-time employee should likewise be expected to work every second weekend. Effective scheduling requires flexibility of part-time personnel, and it is not possible to schedule effectively by working around part-time employees who are available only for certain limited times.

3) *Vacation.* Vacations should be requested, approved, and scheduled in advance, preferably with at least 30 days' notice so that a complete work schedule can always be generated three to four weeks in advance of the time it is to apply, and so that summer replacements or other temporary help can be arranged to help cover periods of peak vacation.

4) *Sick time.* Any employee using consecutive sick days should be required to produce a physician's certification after a limited amount of time off, perhaps two days or certainly no more than three days. This places a slight amount of pressure on the inappropriate use of sick time and helps keep the use of consecutive sick days to a minimum.

5) *Hiring for off shifts.* Departmental hiring should concentrate primarily on acquiring personnel for the off shifts (evenings and nights). The majority of new and potential employees prefer the day shift, and the institution will usually have more persons who are willing to work days than are needed. If a department hires essentially for the second and third shifts as a condition of employment, employees can then be given the option of moving up to the day shift as openings occur.

6) *Holidays.* An employee who earns a holiday by working on a holiday itself should be required to take that earned day off within a reasonable time, for instance, two weeks before or after the occurrence of the actual holiday. If the compensating holiday has not been taken within the required period, the department should schedule this day off at the department's convenience. To preserve the ability to continue scheduling time three to four weeks ahead of time, the department cannot have unexpected "holidays" occurring on a daily basis.

7) *Weekend sick call* Employees who call in sick when scheduled for weekend work should be rescheduled to work the following weekend. This practice tends to reduce weekend sick calls because the people who do so do not avoid weekend work.

8) *Central scheduling.* When possible or practical, all scheduling for the department should be done centrally by a single individual. This is the best way to maintain consistency of approach and overall fairness and to keep personnel pressures and personality considerations out of scheduling. Central scheduling will also minimize the honoring of individual requests for schedule changes and time off.

9) *Shift switching.* All instances of shift switching (two employees mutually agreeing to trade with each other and work each other's shifts) should be done only with the knowledge of the scheduler and the knowledge and permission of the supervisor or supervisors involved. Full knowledge and approval of those responsible for staffing and scheduling help assure that the persons switching are appropriate to the assignments and encourage the switching parties both to fulfill the arrangement. It may also be helpful to institute a buddy system under which various employees are paired for the purpose of switching with each other when appropriate.

10) *Supplement core staff with call-in staff.* The basic core staff established for each unit or department should be augmented with per diem or optional staff during periods of increased workload. This is best approached through the development of a working list of per diem call-in staff who can, within reason, be relied upon to work when needed. This use of per diem or optional staff helps to preserve staffing flexibility while avoiding built-in overstaffing.

Cyclical Scheduling

The principle underlying cyclical scheduling is a repeating work pattern; everyone working on such a schedule has to work the same combination of days on and days off. The scheduling process can be considerably simplified because of the repeating pattern. For instance, consider the schedule of Exhibit 9-1, a four-week schedule for four full-time nurses.

This schedule provides alternate weekends off (0 = day off), splits the other days off, and achieves a core staff of two on weekend days and at least three on weekdays. The minimum number of consecutive days worked (the "work stretch") is three in every case and the maximum is four. Every nurse is working exactly the same schedule, but not at the same time. That is, nurse #1's second week is the same as nurse #2's first week; nurse #1's third week is the same as nurse #3's first week; and nurse #1's fourth week is the same

Exhibit 9-1 Four-Week Schedule:
Four Full-Time Nurses

	S	M	T	W	T	F	S	S	M	T	W	T	F	S	S	M	T	W	T	F	S	S	M	T	W	T	F	S
Nurse #1	O				O				O					O	O					O				O				O
Nurse #2		O					O	O					O				O				O	O				O		
Nurse #3	O					O				O				O	O				O				O					O
Nurse #4			O				O	O				O				O					O	O					O	

(O = Day Off)

as nurse #4's first week. Similarly, nurse #2's schedule consists of the first weeks of each of the other nurses' schedules in this order: nurse #2, nurse #3, nurse #4, nurse #1. This schedule could thus be abbreviated as illustrated in Exhibit 9-2.

According to Exhibit 9-2:

- Nurse 1's schedule would be weeks 1, 2, 3, and 4.
- Nurse 2's schedule would be weeks 2, 3, 4, and 1.
- Nurse 3's schedule would be weeks 3, 4, 1, and 2.
- Nurse 4's schedule would be weeks 4, 1, 2, and 3.

Exhibit 9-2 Abbreviated Four-Week Schedule:
Four Full-Time Nurses

	S	M	T	W	T	F	S
Week #1	O				O		
Week #2		O					O
Week #3	O					O	
Week #4			O				O

(O = Day Off)

In a similar manner a three-nurse schedule which provides for every third weekend off can be generated, as illustrated in Exhibit 9-3 under this schedule:

- Nurse 1's schedule would be weeks 1, 2, 3, and then repeat.
- Nurse 2's schedule would be weeks 2, 3, 1, and then repeat.
- Nurse 3's schedule would be weeks 3, 1, 2, and then repeat.

A modification of the schedule of Exhibit 9-3 can be used to generate a similar schedule for four nurses which provides them with every third weekend off. The minimum cycle length would be 12 weeks; each nurse would move progressively through the 12-week cycle and repeat. However, the addition of a fourth person not only complicates the problem by lengthening the basic cycle but also results in a varying amount of excess staff during each week. Therefore, the practice of allowing every third weekend off works best when personnel exist in multiples of three.

The relationship between weekend coverage policy and minimum core staff is clearly identifiable. Under an alternate weekends off arrangement, the required number of positions is at least twice as many as are needed on any one weekend (since half of the staff is off each weekend). If staff members have every third weekend off, the minimum staff required consists of at least one-and-one-half times the required weekend coverage.

Shift Rotation

In patient care departments, core staff is defined as the minimum number of each skill level required to render proper patient care. For a nursing unit, core staff is normally expressed as a minimum number of registered nurses, licensed practical nurses, nursing aides or assistants, and perhaps unit

---

Exhibit 9-3 Abbreviated Three-Week Schedule: Three Full-Time Nurses

	S	M	T	W	T	F	S
Week #1		O				O	
Week #2			O				O
Week #3	O				O		

(O = Day Off)

secretaries for each shift. The required minimums are often different for weekdays and weekend days. For example, the staffing pattern for a 35-bed medical/surgical unit might appear as in Exhibit 9-4.

Exhibit 9-4 Core Staff for 35-Bed Medical/Surgical Unit

Days

	Weekdays	Weekends
RN	5	3
LPN	3	3
Assistant	3	3
Total	11	9

Evenings

	Weekdays	Weekends
RN	1	1
LPN	3	3
Assistant	3	3
Total	7	7

Nights

	Weekdays	Weekends
RN	1	1
LPN	2	2
Assistant	2	2
Total	5	5

One of the objects of the cyclical schedule is to provide at least core staff for every shift without committing injustices to any of the staff. However, there are often problems in locating sufficient staff who are willing to work regular evening and night shift assignments. Consequently, many institutions resort to some form of shift rotation. The precise form of this rotation can vary, but typical philosophies of shift rotation are:

1. Day personnel must work one month of nights in a year.
2. Day personnel must rotate to evenings the equivalent of one week out of four.

   - Evening rotation is required for five consecutive days in a four-week period; or,
   - Evening rotation is required a day at a time in a week, the total of such being equivalent to one week of evenings out of four weeks.

Once shift rotation is considered the possible combinations of staff and shift assignments are practically endless. However, once a practical, repeatable cycle is established, it is a matter of plugging names into the appropriate slots according to whose turn it is to work what shift.

In the development of staffing standards, techniques such as patient classification systems are available to determine the hours per patient day of nursing care required. Further, such techniques also deal with the mix of nursing skills (RNs and others) that may be required and also split the required hours per patient day by shift. For example, a staffing standard for a nursing unit of 4.8 hours per patient day may break down to 2.5 hours on the day shift, 1.5 hours on the evening shift, and 0.8 hours on the night shift.

In larger departments such as nursing service, where there is likely to be the most concern for complete scheduled coverage, scheduling is most likely to be done centrally or perhaps even by computer with minimal judgmental human intervention. In such circumstances the primary concern of the supervisor or other scheduler is not the systematic plugging of names into time slots but the consistent application of the policies that guide the scheduling process and govern the handling of deviations and exceptions.

Floats: A Safety Valve

As previously mentioned, core staff is that staff required to fulfill the basic responsibilities of the department, or, in the case of a nursing unit, to deliver proper patient care under conditions of normal census. If work activity increases, or if census or the average case severity increases in a given nursing unit, it may be advisable to "float" extra personnel into the area. Also, vacation time or greater-than-normal sick time may also suggest the occasional use of float personnel.

In a sizeable department (primarily the department of nursing service) it frequently makes sense to organize a central "float pool" through which many of the day-to-day variations in staffing among the various units can be smoothed. Certainly nursing personnel in every unit do not take vacations at the same time; neither do all nursing units experience the same levels of sick calls at the same time. However, in a department as large as nursing in a medium to large hospital, one can be assured that a given number of nurses will be on vacation at any time and that a given average number of nurses will likely be ill on any particular day.

A float pool is generally established as a cost center in its own right within the department of nursing service. The persons assigned to the float pool (often a predetermined number of all skills, RNs, LPNs, nursing assistants and unit secretaries) are employed specifically for the purpose of floating from one unit to another on a day-to-day or week-to-week basis as they may be needed. A properly organized float pool can provide sick time and vacation relief for a nursing department far more economically than can be done by staffing each unit to provide the same flexibility.

PART-TIME EMPLOYEES: OBVIOUS ADVANTAGES AND HIDDEN DRAWBACKS

It has long been a common practice in health care institutions to make considerable use of part-time employees. Indeed, it often makes good business sense to use part-time employees to cover periods when help is needed but needed only to an extent that is less than a full-time position (such as straight evening coverage for a function that must be staffed until 9:00 PM, or Saturday and Sunday coverage for a single position). As suggested in parts of the preceding discussion, the use of part-time employees continues to enhance an institution's ability to staff for extended work weeks or for complete scheduled coverage. Also, at times when certain needed skills are in short supply it has made sense to concede to desires of available workers for part-time work only, and to recognize that it is better to staff some positions with combinations of part-time employees than not to staff them at all.

However, the supervisor should think twice before readily conceding to employees' and applicants' requests for job sharing and other split-position arrangements, and before deciding to cover any full-time need with a combination of part-time employees. This precaution is advanced because of a number of problems associated with part-time employees, including:

- When a full-time requirement is covered by multiple employees, for example, one full-time position filled by two part-time employees, work continuity can suffer. Continuity and productivity both suffer when it becomes necessary to absorb the effects of start-up and prepare-to-stop activities of two employees. On the average something is lost; because of more frequently occurring starts and stops and longer absences from the job by each employee, the two employees covering the position are up to speed—that is, are at their most productive—for less total time than one employee would be.

- When a full-time position is covered by two people the communications requirements relative to the job are essentially doubled. Two people must know all that goes on regarding the job, and all other persons working relative to this position must cultivate and maintain two communicating relationships instead of one. From the supervisor's point of view, two persons must be communicated with instead of one, very nearly doubling the effort necessary to maintain one-to-one relationships with employees.

- Many personnel-related costs are essentially doubled—recruiting, interviewing and all else involved in the employment process, pre-employment physical examinations, employee orientation, and the like. In terms of the costs of acquiring and maintaining employees, a single part-time employee absorbs fully as much cost as a full-time employee.

- Some employee benefit costs are increased by increased part-time employment. Many health institutions have long provided full health insurance coverage for part-time employees who regularly work at a certain level, for example, 20 hours or more per week. The cost to the institution of such benefits is the same for a part-time employee as it is for a full-time employee.

- Many of the tasks at or near the heart of the supervisor's job are increased in difficulty and frequency. When two part-time employees fill one full-time slot, the supervisor has two communicating relationships to maintain, two performance evaluations to do, two times the employee-related paperwork to contend with, and the potential for twice as many people problems.

As should also be the case with flextime and other nonconventional work schedule options, the supervisor's key consideration in deciding on the use of part-time employees should be that of business need—the clear furthering of the objectives of the institution. Even when it is obvious that a significant percentage of part-time employment would lend itself to economical staffing with full coverage, this advantage is at least partly offset by the supervisory work inherent in the larger work group and the higher cost of acquiring and maintaining the greater number of employees. When the business need suggests a full-time employee, the supervisor should be cautious about giving ground in the direction of filling such a position with a combination of part-time employees.

NONCONVENTIONAL WORK SCHEDULES

The 40-hour work week has been a practice in many industries for decades. This basic work week was solidified in the Fair Labor Standards Act of 1938 when 40 hours was established as a limit beyond which overtime premium was to be paid. The majority of employees still work a basic work week of 35 to 40 hours spread evenly over five days per week. In recent years, however, various types of nonconventional work schedules have emerged.

Types of Nonconventional Schedules

1) *Compressed work week.* The compressed work week ordinarily consists of the customary 35 to 40 total hours, but these hours are worked in fewer than five days. For example: a critical care nursing unit in a medium-sized hospital is staffed with rotating personnel most of whom work four 10-hour days each week; a large hospital's information systems department, an around-the-clock operation, has computer operators on a weekly schedule of three 12-hour days (for actual operations) followed by a single four-hour shift (for related paperwork and continuing education) over a four-day span; in another critical care unit, nurses work three consecutive 12-hour days to comprise a basic 36-hour work week.

The compressed work week has been applied, both successfully and unsuccessfully, in a variety of work settings.

2) *Total flextime.* Under a total flextime arrangement employees may come and go as they please; they need only to put in whatever total hours are required of them for the work week (usually 35 to 40). They are of course required to accomplish the work expected of them.

Total flextime is impractical for all employees except for those rare individuals whose work is so totally independent of the work of others as to be appropriately accomplished at any time at all. Also, even when total flextime may appear appropriate within a work group, it can present problems or at least perceptions of problems in that it is vulnerable enough to potential abuses to appear to be uncontrollable.

3) *Limited flextime.* Limited flextime allows workers the option of establishing their own starting and quitting times on the condition that they

be present for a specified block of time that may be relatively broad or narrow. Two examples:

- In one personnel department the employment office is open to the public from 9:00 AM to 4:00 PM. The employees of this office, normally putting in an 8 ½ hour day, can alter their starting and quitting times as they choose as long as they put in the 8 ½ hours to include the 9:00 AM to 4:00 PM time block. Some may choose to work a steady 9:00 AM to 5:30 PM time block; some may choose to work a steady 7:30 AM to 4:00 PM; some may choose to vary from day to day as they wish.
- An accounting department allows its employees to establish their own starting and quitting times as long as they are all present between 11:00 AM and 2:00 PM on most work days. The exception to this is a requirement that they all be present from 9:00 AM to 4:00 PM during the week of the monthly closing of the books. So long as they work these required blocks of time, the accounting employees may work longer or shorter days at their option while putting in 40 hours each week.

4) *Team flextime.* Under the team flextime concept all employees of a department or clearly designated team agree on their starting and quitting times as a group. This arrangement has been particularly popular with tightly unified work groups, such as operating room teams who may choose to arrange their schedule around surgeons' operating practices.

5) *Job sharing.* Job sharing consists of two or more people working part-time and mutually arranging their schedules so as to fill one single position. The most common job-sharing situations involve two part-time employees filling one full-time position. One pertinent example would be the position of department secretary in the department of surgery in a particular hospital; this position is filled by two half-time employees who each work alternating weeks of three days and two days.

The Growing Role of Nonconventional Work Schedules

Nonconventional work schedules are growing in popularity with many employees, and it is becoming increasingly clear that there are instances in which such schedules may be in the best interest of institutions. Encouraging nonconventional work schedules are:

- the family requirements of workers who are part of two-career families;
- the declining numbers of people with some critically needed skills, which causes organizations to entice people with favorable work schedules;

- changing lifestyles that lead to the desire for more time for leisure and personal pursuits.

The frequently expressed doubts of many supervisors concerning nonconventional work schedules seem to spring from:

- their longstanding familiarity with conventional eight-hour per day, five-day per week practices;
- their hesitancy to go contrary to what everyone else is doing;
- their understandable fear of the unknown, of new problems they believe may be associated with such dramatic changes in practice.

However, more than a few organizations have discovered that nonconventional work schedules have:

- helped improve productivity;
- permitted improved utilization of facilities and equipment;
- helped in recruiting and retaining employees in certain skills that have been in short supply.

All of the nonconventional work schedule variations have advantages and disadvantages, and none is fully appropriate to all departments and in all situations. The supervisor must achieve a balance between legitimate business needs and the needs and desires of employees.

The Department Supervisor's Perspective

The supervisor must consider with great care the possible adoption of a nonconventional work schedule. Within some departments and functions, longer shifts can lead to increased employee tension and fatigue and thus to increased errors. Also within some departments and functions, excessive freedom to establish one's own starting and quitting times can leave a function overstaffed when fewer people are required and understaffed when more are needed. And as with any approach that gives people more autonomy than they are accustomed to, there may be occasional employees who abuse the privileges.

However, if a nonconventional work schedule appears appropriate to the department's situation, the supervisor could conceivably spend considerably less time dealing with tardiness and attendance problems and also spend less time dealing with time off and other requests for juggled schedules. Nonconventional work schedules are obviously not for every department and every worker. Many people are solidly adjusted to the eight-hour day and five-day week and may choose not to disrupt this pattern even if given the chance.

Thus when any nonconventional work schedule is proposed or seriously considered, the supervisor should make every effort to determine:

- Can all of the functions of the department be adequately covered under the proposed approach?
- Will quality and quantity of service be maintained or improved under the proposed approach?
- Are the majority of employees in favor of the approach or at least willing to give it a fair trial?

If a negative answer develops regarding any of the foregoing questions, the supervisor should perhaps drop the proposal or at least first work to overcome the apparent problems. It makes little sense to go forward on employee preferences and desires alone if there is not a definite business advantage to the proposed change. However, it is not appropriate to attempt to force a change to a nonconventional work schedule on the basis of business advantage alone if doing so would prove upsetting to employees.

If one employee requests a flextime arrangement the supervisor must then consider: "If all of my employees ask me for the same arrangement, would the staffing needs of the department allow me to grant the request?" In short, if any particular flextime arrangement cannot be granted for all of a group, consistency of employee treatment suggests that it cannot be granted for just one or a few.

IT ALL BEGINS WITH A STAFFING STANDARD

The staffing part of staffing and scheduling—the determination of how many people of what skills are needed to do the work—comes first. The starting point, the staffing standard, is often no more than an indication of traditional output or what has worked in the past. Such rough staffing guidelines are generally indefensible for some purposes, but nevertheless a broad guide is often better than none. For effective staffing and scheduling, every department needs an engineered staffing standard that can be reasonably defended under most conditions.

The determination of a staffing standard usually lies beyond the supervisor's power, but if the development of a standard is properly pursued the supervisor will have active input in the process. And although a staffing standard may occasionally be seen as a drawback in that it might be applied to remove supposed overstaffing, the standard can apply in the opposite direction: A credible, defensible, verifiable staffing standard provides the supervisor's best possible justification for more staff when such is required.

In summary, staffing and scheduling for optimum productivity requires:

- that staffing standards, or at least targets, be established;
- that policies be established to facilitate the consistent pursuit of effective staffing and scheduling;
- that there be a comprehensive employee relations program to help assure that people produce not because they are forced to but because they want to.

NOTE

1. Clifford Neely, "Hospital Economic Forecast," *Hospitals* 58 (13), July 1, 1984, p. 78.

Chapter 10

Keeping Overtime under Control

By losing present time we lose all time.

Old Proverb

Chapter Objectives

- Review the portions of the Fair Labor Standards Act that define overtime and specify its methods of compensation.
- Place overtime into proper perspective as a cost factor.
- Identify the common causes of overtime.
- Develop suggested approaches for supervisory control of overtime.
- Identify means of overcoming the problems commonly encountered in attempting to control overtime.

OVERTIME AND THE LEGAL WORK WEEK

As defined within the lengthy text of the Fair Labor Standards Act (FLSA), the work week:

- is a regularly recurring period of 168 hours;
- consists of seven consecutive 24-hour periods;
- can be designated as beginning at any hour on any day of the week;
- can apply to all employees of the organization, or different work weeks can be established for different groups of employees[1].

Under the provisions of the FLSA nonexempt employees are entitled to overtime for hours worked in excess of 40 per work week. This is generally understood in most work organizations. However, in many organizations nonexempt employees are paid overtime on the basis of hours worked in excess of 8 per day or 40 per week. This practice, paying overtime for more than 8 hours in a day as well as 40 hours in a week, is in some places so widespread that many persons have assumed that overtime payment for hours in excess of 8 in a day is part of the legal requirement. Such is not the case; although many organizations choose to pay overtime for hours in excess of 8 in a day, thus making overtime pay available to persons who work less than full time or who experience absences during the work week, the legal requirement of FLSA addresses only hours worked in excess of 40 in a week.

Under a special provision in FLSA, health care institutions are allowed to use a work period of 14 days instead of a 7-day work week.[2] The expression of this practice is the so-called "8-and-80 exemption" found in some health care institutions. When the 8-and-80 exemption is in place, overtime must be paid for hours worked in excess of 8 in a day or 80 in a 14-day period. It should be stressed that although the 8-in-a-day threshold does not exist in the government's treatment of the 7-day work week, the 8-in-a-day threshold is a legal requirement under the 8-and-80 exemption. A health care organization that adopts the 8-and-80 exemption must do so with the intent of retaining it permanently or at least for a substantial period of time. The organization cannot change back and forth between the 8-and-80 and the normal 7-day work week, since doing so will, at least in terms of perceptions and very often in fact, be taken as intended to avoid the payment of overtime.

All of the overtime referred to in FLSA—hours in excess of 40 in a normal 7-day work week, or hours in excess of 8 per day or 80 hours total in a 14-day period—must be paid at time-and-one-half the employee's regular rate.[3] This regular rate is not simply an employee's base rate of pay; in addition to including the employee's base rate it also includes other earned amounts, such as shift differential, call-in pay, and certain forms of on-call pay, that the employee receives for performing services during the applicable time period. In other words, an employee's regular rate for a given time period is an average hourly rate based on all elements of earnings associated with the employee's normal work period.

Impact of Different Work Weeks

It has already been noted that FLSA allows employers to establish the work week as beginning at any hour of any day of the week. The most prevailing work weeks found within the health care setting are Monday through Sunday and Sunday through Saturday (that is, a 168-hour period beginning and ending at midnight Sunday or at midnight Saturday). A few health institutions utilize other work weeks—Wednesday through Tuesday is occasionally used—and some health care organizations, working under an organization-wide 8-and-80 exemption, average employees' hours over a two-week period. The organization's definition of the work week, as well as the organization's scheduling practices and method of overtime payment, can have a definite impact on overtime costs.

Exhibit 10-1 shows three variations of a simple two-week schedule assembled under different work week definitions. Schedule A, based on a Monday through Sunday work week, shows four days worked during week one and six days worked in week two. Under the ordinary requirement of the FLSA for overtime to be paid for hours in excess of 40 in a week, this schedule automatically incurs overtime payment during the second week.

Schedule B represents the same schedule as Schedule A but applies to a Sunday through Saturday work week. This schedule shows five work days in each week and thus incurs no overtime. Likewise Schedule C, based on a Wednesday through Tuesday work week, also incurs no overtime.

Exhibit 10-2 shows the work week definition when combined with an organization's policy of scheduling no split days off (that is, a requirement that an employee's two days off each week will always be two consecutive days). Under these conditions the Sunday through Saturday work week (Schedule B of Exhibit 10-2) incurs overtime costs, but the other two schedules do not.

Notice the likely effect of having the 8-and-80 exemption in place: If overtime were to be computed on the excess of hours over those worked on ten normal shifts in a two-week period, all of the potential overtime problems in the schedules of Exhibits 10-1 and 10-2 are eliminated. In general, the two-week averaging of the 8-and-80 exemption tends to provide managers with more scheduling flexibility.

In some circumstances it is possible to apply the 8-and-80 exemption to specific individuals or specifically defined groups of employees while not applying it to the organization as a whole. However, such special cases must

Exhibit 10-1 Scheduling under Different Work Week Definitions

Schedule A

	M	T	W	T	F	S	S
Week #1	O					O	O
Week #2				O			

Schedule B

	S	M	T	W	T	F	S
Week #1		O					O
Week #2	O				O		

Schedule C

	W	T	F	S	S	M	T
Week #1				O	O		
Week #2		O				O	

(O = Day Off)

be agreed to in writing by employees and organization alike and it must be clearly demonstrated that the arrangement is to both the benefit of the organization and the convenience of the employee and that it does not avoid paying the employee any earned time. For example, consider an organization with a defined Sunday through Saturday work week and an employee working according to Schedule B of Exhibit 10-2. Assume that this schedule is strongly preferred by the employee as a normal schedule, and further that this schedule works for the convenience of the organization. However, this schedule places four days in one work week and six days in the other. To resolve this problem, the organization and the employees can jointly agree

Exhibit 10-2 Scheduling under Different Work Week Definitions
(No Split Days Off)

Schedule A

	M	T	W	T	F	S	S
Week #1						O	O
Week #2				O	O		

Schedule B

	S	M	T	W	T	F	S
Week #1							O
Week #2	O				O	O	

Schedule C

	W	T	F	S	S	M	T
Week #1				O	O		
Week #2		O	O				

(O = Day Off)

---

to a documented exception to the rule of FLSA and apply the 8-and-80 exemption in this situation.

The individual supervisor will generally have little influence on determining the organization's work week or on whether the mode of overtime payment will be based on 40 hours or on an organization-wide 8-and-80 policy. However, the supervisor can, and certainly should, be aware of the scheduling limitations imposed by the organization's work week definition, and should likewise be aware of the mode of overtime payment, and schedule within all of these limitations in a manner that avoids building automatic overtime into employees' work schedules.

OVERTIME AS A COST FACTOR

The increasing emphasis on the need for cost containment will undoubtedly increase the pressure on supervisors to control overtime and to justify economically all of the overtime that is used. Overtime has long been viewed in different ways by managers in health care organizations. Some supervisors and managers consider some amount of overtime to be essential and recognize it as less costly than adding more staff for certain occasional needs. Others behave as though they view overtime as a form of reward to be extended to the department's better employees, and others appear to view overtime as an unnecessary expense to be avoided at all times.

Certainly the department that uses too much overtime—and "too much" can be difficult to define—is going to have cost problems. However, there may also be a problem (a different problem, but just as or even more severe) in the department that never uses overtime. It is highly probable that a department that never uses overtime is overstaffed.

In most departments some overtime may at times be necessary; sometimes it is the best way to cover certain needs. However, overtime is inherently costly and its use can easily get out of hand.

One element of cost is obvious: The person who is on overtime is receiving 50 percent more pay for those hours than an equivalently paid employee who is doing the same work during nonovertime hours. Nevertheless, the cost of overtime is often less than the cost of hiring more staff to cover the needs because of the additional elements of cost associated with employment.

An employee working regular, nonpremium hours earns, in addition to a base rate of pay, benefits that cost an additional 30 to 40 percent of base pay (health insurance, life insurance, sick time, holidays, and vacation), but an employee working overtime does not ordinarily accrue additional benefits while working on premium time. Thus the cost gap between an employee on overtime and a new employee is considerably narrowed. Also, the acquisition of a new employee is subject to the costs of recruiting, hiring, and training. Although an organization-specific cost analysis would have to be done on a case-by-case basis, it is generally safe to say that when benefit costs are added to other elements of cost associated with employment, paying for an added employee can often be more costly than paying overtime to an existing employee. Although added long-term requirements should be subject to careful scrutiny and cost analysis to determine the point at which costs may break even, for short-term, infrequent, or sporadic requirements, it is usually more cost effective to ask existing employees to work overtime. The control of overtime requires constant balancing of legitimate needs against resources available. Since legitimate short-term needs are often best met through the use of overtime, one can never say that overtime is always bad.

CAUSES OF OVERTIME

The causes of overtime are many and varied, but within the organization that may be experiencing excessive overtime use these causes often include all or most of the following:

- Variations in workload. The variations in workload most often giving rise to overtime are those due to unexpected changes in demand, unanticipated alterations in deadlines, and genuine emergency situations. Since variations of this nature are not predictable, overtime is often the only recourse.
- Absenteeism. In many departments there is a demonstrable, direct relationship between employee absenteeism and the need for overtime; absenteeism increases and the requests for overtime increase (refer to Chapter 11, Reducing and Controlling Absenteeism).
- Acceptance of substandard performance. An attitude of passivity sometimes permeates supervision and work force alike. All parties come to accept that work not accomplished on regular time will be done on overtime, and thus by default a practice develops of rewarding substandard performance.
- General acceptance of overtime as a normal practice rather than an exception. If the prevailing attitude is that overtime has always been used to catch up or make up, then overtime always will be used to catch up and make up.
- Lack of supervisor accountability. If the supervisor does not have to answer directly to his or her superior for the use of overtime without particular concern for its costs, this leads to the acceptance of overtime as normal and less likely to be seen as a recourse to handle true exceptions.
- Rigid scheduling practices. When the supervisor or scheduler is constrained so severely by scheduling practices as to be unable to schedule without causing overtime in cyclical schedules, an implied guarantee of overtime has been extended to elements of the work force. Built-in overtime, and indeed all forms of guaranteed overtime, undermine the basic purposes of overtime and again lead toward its acceptance as a normal practice.
- Bargaining unit work rules. Various labor contracts state that only certain classifications of employees can do certain kinds of work. Often under such rules, the logical persons to meet unforeseen requirements, such as part-time employees who could have their hours temporarily increased, are prevented from being used appropriately because the con-

tract may state, for example, that overtime must be offered first to full-time employees in order of seniority.

- Inappropriate or insufficient equipment and inefficient physical work area. Physical conditions that increase worker fatigue or that impede the efficient performance of work often make it necessary to catch up using overtime. When it comes to productivity, an employee can be only as efficient as the equipment and the work environment will allow.

A certain common-sense logic suggests that overtime is often the cleanest, most reasonable way of coping with emergency situations and meeting necessary nonrecurring needs. Applied according to this logic, occasional overtime is generally supportive of sustained productivity. However, regular overtime—constant overtime for some workers as a permanent or semipermanent condition—can be counterproductive. In the extreme, increases in overtime can lead to decreased job satisfaction, increased fatigue, and decreased productivity. Decreased job satisfaction and increased fatigue will often lead to increased absenteeism; increased absenteeism and decreased productivity can in turn lead to a more intensified need for output. This intensified need for output will then be a direct stimulus to the continued use of overtime. Thus continuing overtime is itself one of the forces that often causes more overtime to be worked.

At its worst, continuing overtime is costly, disruptive, and counterproductive. Even at its best, continuing overtime becomes part of the employee's "normal" time available for doing work. As Parkinson stated years ago, "Work expands so as to fill the time availble for its completion."[4] Thus under conditions of continual overtime, the view of the work week gradually broadens until this extended week is seen as the normal time frame within which one's work is to be done.

TOWARD CONTROL OF OVERTIME

The general approaches available to the supervisor for the control of overtime are:

1) *Regulate demand.* In some departments—and certainly there are a number of functions within a health care institution to which this cannot apply—it is possible to take action that regulates the demand on the department's services. The approaches available for the regulation of demand include:

- Working on a reservation or appointment basis. This is probably the most common means of smoothing demand. Simply stated, people who must come to the department for service are given specific appointments.

The intent is to spread the arrival of work as uniformly as possible over the work day to minimize the possibility of periods of excess activity and periods of inactivity.

- Promoting low-demand periods. Making it known, for example, that waiting time at the cashier's office is minimal or nonexistent after 3:00 PM, or that cafeteria lines are shortest between 11:30 AM and 12 noon and 1:00 and 1:30 PM, can cause some users to rearrange their use of these facilities to take advantage of faster service.
- Complementary scheduling. When two or more groups of people are usually calling upon the same service and when access to that service can be controlled for some of these would-be users, it is often possible to schedule certain kinds of users into certain time periods. Consider, for example, an electrocardiography unit that services both inpatients and outpatients on an emergency basis as well as a scheduled basis, and experiences an extremely high volume of outpatient work during the two or three morning hours when the outpatient department's clinics are operating. Inpatient services, which may be a significant part of the workload, may be scheduled for only those hours during which the clinics are not open, thus assuring a measurable movement in workload away from the busiest time to a time when more capacity should be available.

In general, any steps that can be taken to regulate demand—to smooth the arrival of work into the department so that it is better distributed throughout the work day—will serve to decrease the need for overtime. In many instances demand regulation can help avoid circumstances under which, for example, unused capacity exists in a department for the larger part of the day but then overtime becomes necessary because a disproportionate amount arrives in a peak during the latter part of the shift.

2) *Analyze and improve staffing practices.* Among the steps the supervisor can consider to improve the department's staffing practices and thus help reduce excessive overtime are:

- cross-training employees of equivalent skill and grade in each others' jobs, making it possible to cover more readily for absent employees with employees who may have the time;
- using floats as appropriate, personnel from the department's float pool if such exists;
- utilizing the services of per diem or optional staff who will work an occasional day or a few hours when called;
- increasing the hours of selected part-time employees to cover nonrecurring emergency needs;

- constantly reevaluating the department's scheduling practices to assure that as much as possible these practices recognize the reality of the department's staffing circumstances.

3) *Analyze and improve work methods.* Ineffective work methods, inadequate operating procedures, ineffective, obsolete, or otherwise inappropriate equipment, inefficient workplace layout—all of these tend to depress productivity and thus increase the pressure for overtime. Look closely at backlogs of work and bottleneck situations that seem to require periodic overtime to bring them into line (refer to Chapter 8, Methods Improvement).

4) *Control absenteeism.* As suggested earlier, more often than not there is a direct relationship between the department's level of absenteeism and the amount of overtime worked. To address absenteeism directly is to address directly the problem of excess overtime as well (refer to Chapter 11, Reducing and Controlling Absenteeism).

5) *Supervise responsibly.* Supervising responsibly is to consider oneself as accountable for the level of overtime usage in the department. Acceptance of this accountability suggests a thorough, rational approach to the examination of each instance of possible overtime. When possible overtime need arises, check first to determine whether the work can be postponed, reassigned to staff who are on hand, or accomplished by faster, more efficient means. If any of these can be done, make the appropriate arrangements.

If the work cannot be postponed or reassigned or accomplished by other means, check for:

- available part-time employees or float personnel, or available call-in help;
- available full-time staff who have been absent part of the week. Under the strict FLSA requirement of overtime for over 40 hours—and in the absence of an organizational policy for overtime for more than 8 hours in a day—staff who have been absent for part of a week are often willing to make up all or part of the balance of the work week by working at their regular rates.

Only upon exhausting all of the foregoing possibilities without resolution should the supervisor approve overtime, and then only consistent with the organization's policy (in some organizations the supervisor is required to obtain the approval of the next higher level of management).

Once approved, overtime should then be performed preferably by some employee other than the incumbent of the position who has perhaps already worked at that job for an entire work day (unless such substitution is forbidden by the provisions of a labor contract). Doing so, accomplishing the overtime with a substitute employee, avoids any possibility of rewarding an employee with overtime pay for failing to accomplish the day's work in the normally expected time. This action should be taken with discretion as the supervisor attempts to differentiate between those occurrences of overtime that are due to substandard performance and those that lie beyond the employee's control.

Finally, for each instance keep an accurate record of the reason for the overtime, the amount of time involved, and the specific staff used to cover the need.

COMMON CONTROL PROBLEMS

From the supervisor's perspective, legal and procedural problems with overtime are most likely to arise out of gaps in one's knowledge of law and policy, out of difficulties with overtime authorization processes, and out of difficulty with time-recording practices.

Knowledge of Law and Policy

The supervisor should know the pertinent parts of the law as embodied in FLSA, and should know whether the basic 40-hour work week or the 8-and-80 exemption is in use in the organization. The supervisor should understand also that if overtime is paid beyond 8 hours a day in a 40-hour week, this is policy and not law. Be fully aware of the organization's defined work week and its impact on scheduling.

Further, know what is included in the calculation of an employee's regular rate and the calculation of overtime. The law states what must be included, but organization policy often includes more than is required by law. For example, if the organization pays overtime for hours in excess of 8 per day or 40 in a week, then sick time or vacation time used during the work week is actually being counted in determining overtime although this is not required by law.

Know the differences between exempt employees and nonexempt employees. Nonexempt, as applied in defining employee status, means simply that the employee is not exempt from, that is, is covered by, the overtime requirements of FLSA. Exempt employees are not covered and do not receive overtime. In defining such employees, FLSA says, in effect, who can be exempt and not who must be exempt. For example, most registered nurses can be considered as exempt employees because they generally fit the definition of professional contained in the law. However, in the majority of health care organizations registered nurses are treated as nonexempt employees in that they are paid for overtime work. In terms of who is paid overtime and who is not, FLSA specifies who must be paid overtime. However, others can be paid overtime and in many organizations are paid overtime. In this regard the law requires only that the established practices of the organization be consistently applied.

Overtime Authorization

Supervisors often experience problems with the authorization of overtime. Most organizations' systems call for overtime approval usually in advance of the overtime being worked. However, because of emergency situations advance approval is not always possible, and employees who may be put in the position of having to judge for themselves should know the ground rules.

A common process, embodied in one hospital's overtime pay guidelines, includes the following regarding overtime authorization:

1. Scheduled (anticipated) overtime should be approved in advance by the department supervisor.
2. Unscheduled overtime should be handled as follows:

   - An employee who determines that it may be necessary to work beyond the assigned shift must make a good faith effort to obtain the department supervisor's approval.
   - Unscheduled overtime worked without advance authorization should be reviewed for approval on a daily basis. The department supervisor should initial the time record to indicate approval.
   - Overtime payment should not be permitted to result solely from employees' card-punching practices. Employees not engaged in overtime work should punch in and out according to timekeeping policies.

Time Recording Practices

Most organizations have policies that regulate employees' punching in and punching out within a certain range of time on either side of starting and quitting time. For example, in one organization the rule may be: The employee is to punch in not earlier than ten minutes before the start of the shift and not later than ten minutes after the end of the shift. Another policy commonly encountered requires that employees punch in and out within six minutes (0.1 hours) on either side of starting and quitting time.

The organization is in a position of vulnerability if employees punch in too long a time before the start of the shift or punch out too long a time after the end of the shift. Unfortunately, however, it is not possible to say with universality how long constitutes too long. Ordinarily the organization's payroll department will not compensate for so-called "casual" overtime in small amounts without signed approval, but this does not reduce the organization's vulnerability. Common sense should suggest that a few minutes spent by an employee on the premises before or after the shift need not and would not be included in the hours worked. However, even the small amounts of extra work that some employees do before punching out, although not approved as overtime, are legally compensable at overtime rates under FLSA. An organization's prohibition against overtime work is no protection from legal overtime pay liability, and even a policy to the effect that only requested and authorized overtime will be paid for will not protect the employer. Upon audit by the Department of Labor, more than a few employer organizations have been required to pay retroactively for significant accumulations of so-called casual overtime.

CONSTANT VISIBILITY

A significant part of the control of overtime consists of maintaining the topic in a position of prominence and paying attention to its importance. One way of keeping overtime visible to the department is to publicize, on a regular monthly basis, the department's performance against budget in its use of overtime. If overtime is not a separately budgeted item (although in most organizations it is that), then at budget preparation time the supervisor should suggest strongly that overtime be made a budget subaccount of its own and that actual overtime be reported back against budgeted overtime on the regular budget-reporting cycle.

Another method for keeping the overtime issue visible involves the use of an organization-wide overtime committee. The experience of one organization proved interesting, and since the approach was not particularly unique similar results have likely been experienced elsewhere: An overtime committee was first established during a year in which overtime apparently went completely out of control. Consisting of a dozen or more people—administration, finance, and the heads of major departments—the committee wrestled with the causes of overtime and the overtime approval process, and watched overtime usage diminish until it was within budget limits. When the problem went away, the committee began to meet less often and eventually not at all; overtime again rose. However, each time the committee was reconstituted in response to rising overtime, overtime immediately began to track downward. Each time the committee could do no more than it had done before, could recommend no more than had been recommended in the past, and yet each time the amount of visible concern for overtime began to increase, the amount of overtime used throughout the organization began concurrently to decrease. Thus visible attention paid to overtime is often sufficient to impress people with its importance so that they become more careful.

If a department is properly staffed, it will likely experience some overtime needs from time to time. Overtime will always be subject to a certain amount of abuse, abuse that likely will increase if it is not made plain that overtime is subject to constant scrutiny. Even if the problem is resolved periodically, it is likely to recur. The only long-run solution to the control of overtime is an appropriate level of constant attention and active monitoring and control by supervision.

NOTES

1. Richard B. Gallagher and Frank D. Wagner, "Overtime Pay" in *Federal Regulation of Employment Service* (New York: Research Institute of America, 1982), Sec. 29.3.
2. Ibid., Sec. 29.7.
3. Ibid., Sec. 29.12 and 29.13.
4. C. Northcote Parkinson, *Parkinson's Law* (Boston: Houghton Mifflin, 1957), p. 1.

Chapter 11

Reducing and Controlling Absenteeism

It's called absenteeism. In school we called it hooky. Both words describe an illness that sneaks up on you.

Ellis D. Roberts

Chapter Objectives

- Examine the differing perceptions of sick time, and place sick time in perspective as an employee benefit.
- Discuss the general causes of employee absenteeism.
- Establish absenteeism as a continuing problem requiring constant, visible supervisory concern.
- Suggest how the supervisor may go about addressing the problem of employee absenteeism in general and the apparent abuse of sick time in particular.
- Explore the characteristics and advantages and disadvantages of employee-incentive approaches to the control of sick time.

SICK TIME AS A BENEFIT

In most organizations that offer paid sick time to employees, considerably different views will likely exist concerning the uses of this time. In many cases it is attitude that induces some employees to take sick time for granted and thus leads these employees toward excessive absenteeism.

One can argue convincingly, although perhaps not completely, that sick time either is or is not a true benefit in the institution's so-called employee benefits package. However, such arguments turn out to be little more than word play that simply calls into question our definition and concept of benefits. All of the features of the employment relationship that are regarded as benefits are generally recognized as additions to employee compensation. However, each addition to compensation must also be recognized as being one of two distinct kinds:

1) *Entitlements*. These are forms of earned compensation which accrue to the employee by way of some formula or pattern. Once earned, an entitlement belongs to the employee. For example, vacation time is an entitlement—once it is earned it belongs to the employee, and all that remains to be determined is its form of payment (either paid-time-off or cash) and the timing of payment. Likewise, holiday time, earned and credited consistent with the organization's policy for observing legal holidays, is generally an entitlement, as are future pension payments for an employee who has fulfilled the vesting requirements of a retirement plan.

2) *Insurance-type benefits*, consistently distributed among employees according to certain terms of employment, are intended to compensate for some specified conditions only if and when these conditions occur. The purest and most obvious forms of insurance-type benefits are employer-supplied life insurance, health and medical insurance, and disability insurance.

As originally constituted in most organizations, and as still regarded in the majority of work organizations, sick time is provided as the second type of benefit, a form of insurance intended to protect employees from loss of income owing to short-term illness. However, in the minds of many employees sick time is viewed more as an entitlement than as a form of insurance. Sick time is seen by many as earned compensation which, once earned, belongs to the employee and thus should be used (and must be used or it is lost). No doubt this attitude was initially fostered and continually reinforced by organizational policies calling for the granting of so many sick days per employee per year in precisely the same way that vacation and holiday time were allocated. Also, in recent years the widespread view of sick time as an entitlement has been strongly reinforced by the use of sick-time incentive programs that offer employees some form of payment for reducing their consumption of sick time.

Regardless of individual views of sick time as either an entitlement or a form of insurance, however, the true characteristic of sick time and all other benefits lies in the accounting treatment. True entitlements, representing a form of employee earnings, go into the books of the organization as liabilities, obligations that must be paid. When an employee earns so many days of vacation time, that time goes on the books as a liability and must be carried as such in the accounting process. There is no question about the value of those days owing to the employee; the only question is one of how this obligation will be paid, generally as either paid-time-off arranged according to some schedule or as cash equivalent paid upon termination. One way or another, once earned, an entitlement will eventually be paid. Such is not the case with sick time; sick time does not go into the organization's books of account as a liability. Its recording is simply a numerical accounting of the amount of sick time available to each employee. The only time the value of sick time enters the books of account is when a specific amount of expense is recorded for sick time actually used. Thus the most accurate characterization of sick time is as the organization's form of self-insurance protection of its employees against loss of earnings because of short-term illness.

Although assumed by many to be an entitlement, sick time is simply a form of insurance to be used only when needed. And as with any form of insurance, its use must be controlled relative to its cost.

ABSENTEEISM: COST AND CAUSES

According to an estimate early in 1984, work missed by every one of the country's 60.2 million nonfarm workers costs more than $60 apiece per year on the average.[1] Thus an employer of 1,000 people could expect to see a $60,000 annual budget impact of missed time. These same figures suggest that the total financial impact of the time missed by all of the nation's 60.2 million nonfarm workers amounts to $3.6 billion per year.

Other estimates are considerably higher than the foregoing. One source suggests that absenteeism costs American industry as a whole close to $10 billion per year.[2] Another example specific to the level of the health care institution stated that a 1980 year-long study of a midwest hospital noted 182,700 hours of employee absence; at the prevailing average rate of $6.50 per hour, these hours translated into $1,187,550 lost in one year due to employee absence.[3]

Of course, much of the sick time used by employees is taken for legitimate reasons involving personal illness and, as some organization's policies may permit, medical and dental appointments. However, a significant amount of sick time use—absenteeism—is unwarranted and constitutes abuse of sick time privileges. As suggested in the earlier discussion that drew a distinction between those benefits that are entitlements and those that are essentially insurances, sick time is often abused because of the belief—a belief perhaps as strongly held by some managers as by employees—that sick time is an entitlement like vacation rather than a benefit to be applied as needed like health insurance. Also, sick time is often abused because of a general expectation in work organizations that many people will be "out sick" some unknown percentage of the time, and because of an attitude reflected by supervisors conveying the apparent belief that not much can be done about sick time use.

General Causes of Absenteeism

The general causes of absenteeism may be grouped approximately as follows:

1) *Legitimate health problems.* It would at best be extremely difficult to determine for any given organization the proportion of sick time that is taken in response to legitimate health problems. People become ill, and for many short-term illnesses one of the surest forms of treatment is rest. People are injured and require time to recuperate. People who are ill or injured are generally not capable of doing their best work, and in attempting to do so they may endanger patients through errors, impede their own recovery to full effectiveness, perhaps subject others to contamination, and increase the risk of accidents to themselves and others. Since sick time benefits exist to provide income protection in the event of short-term illness or injury, the use of sick time for legitimate health problems is fully appropriate. However, even extending the benefit of the doubt and assuming that half or more of an organization's sick time use is probably legitimate, the typical system will ordinarily include a significant amount of abuse.

2) *Job-related problems.* There is room to ponder whether some job-related problems and circumstances that arise in day-to-day functioning do not perhaps place some employees in a position of feeling that the arbitrary use of a so-called mental health day is the only way to fall back and regroup. There is also room to wonder how much sick time might be consumed by employees who are caught up in unsatisfactory work relationships. Most uses of sick time that appear questionable or inappropriate—inappropriate because they do not involve personal illness or injury—appear to involve the individual's need for temporary escape from job-related problems. Such problems include:

- stress arising from job difficulty, pace, workload, or interpersonal conflict, giving rise to the occasional "mental health day";
- work that is seen as dull, demeaning, distasteful, or lacking interest, variety, or challenge;
- supervision that is seen as unfeeling or uncaring;
- a manager or management group that does not listen and that criticizes but rarely if ever praises or acknowledges contributions.

Also to be considered a job-related problem contributing to sick time use, although not leading employees to seek escape, as might be the case with the aforementioned problems, is the matter of management's attitude toward sick time. If management seems indifferent toward sick time and pays little attention to who is out how often and for what length of time, then management, by omission, is encouraging the use of sick time.

3) *Substance abuse.* Although substance abuse (the abuse of alcohol and drugs, prescription and otherwise) is describable under the general heading of health problems, it is dealt with separately for two reasons: Substance abuse is sufficiently widespread to be considered a problem in its own right; and substance abuse and its effects are usually reflected in job-related problems. There are direct effects on an employee's physical, mental, and emotional health, leading to time lost from work. On the job there are invariably a number of difficulties, perhaps including loss of ambition, diminished energy, impaired coordination and reaction time, impaired judgment, and generally reduced effectiveness, all brought in from the outside by the victim of substance abuse.

4) *Other personal problems and needs.* In this category one may place anything that does not readily fit into the three foregoing categories of problems. Other personal problems and needs might include, for example:

- stress in one's personal life such as that resulting from separation or divorce, problems with children, family members with health problems, or financial or legal difficulties;
- difficulty in maintaining child care arrangements;
- time needed to transact personal business.

The supervisor should be prepared to accept some absence as legitimate and some as inappropriate. However, although with effort the supervisor may be able to gain some insight into the causes of absenteeism, a true reading on how much illness is real and how much is merely convenient will probably remain elusive. Thus one can safely say that a certain level of absenteeism in a department will be a fact of organizational life. Absenteeism cannot be eradicated completely, but it can be controlled. Control, however, requires conscious effort and a visible level of constant attention.

ADDRESSING ABSENTEEISM

In addressing absenteeism the supervisor's initial emphasis should be on prevention, but even though preventive methods will invariably have some positive effect on levels of absenteeism, more will remain to be done. However, well before specifically directed action, such as the application of disciplinary measures, is taken, a preventive posture should be adopted and thereafter maintained by the supervisor.

As noted, any number of different problems may lie behind any instance of employee absence. Studies have shown that there is a definite connection between an employee's working conditions and that employee's attendance: The better the working conditions in the eyes of the employee, the better the employee's attendance will be. Also, it has been established that there is a similar relationship between attendance and the employee's opinion of the supervisor.[4]

Prevention

Much that may affect an employee's job admittedly lies beyond the control of the supervisor. The supervisor nevertheless has primary control over management's treatment of the individual employee. In many cases the group supervisor may be the only member of this otherwise mysterious entity known as management with whom the employee is reasonbly well acquainted. The supervisor may be the only member of management with whom the individual employee has any kind of speaking relationship. Therefore, to the individual employee not only does the supervisor represent management, in a real way the supervisor *is* management to the employee. Thus if the individual employee sees the supervisor as indifferent, uncaring, unconcerned, and perhaps even unavailable most of the time, so also will the employee be likely to regard all of management in this way. One can often go so far as to say that as the employee sees the supervisor, so may he or she also see the entire organization.

At this point it would be possible to insert, with considerable pertinence, a lengthy dissertation on human relations in supervision. However, suffice it to say that since a given amount of absenteeism is inappropriate, and that since much of this inappropriate absenteeism will stem from job-related problems either real or perceived, that the supervisor's style, attitude, and approach have an effect on employee absenteeism. In brief, the beginning of the prevention of absenteeism is a supervisory style and approach that says in effect:

> As supervisor I am here primarily to enable you to get your work done as smoothly and efficiently as possible. I value your participation and I care about you as an individual. Because our efforts are interrelated—you do not work *for* me, but rather *we* work together—I want to help the organization fulfill its employment relationship with you, I want to recognize your successes and your accomplishments, and I want to assist you constructively in becoming more productive if we seem to be faced with difficulties in getting the job done.

Beyond thoughtful, understanding supervision, the prevention of absenteeism next requires that absence be maintained in a position of visibility to employees as a legitimate concern of the department. To do so it is advisable for the supervisor to:

- Assure that each new employee entering the department starts out on the right path, clearly forearmed with expectations regarding attendance and the organization's concern for regular attendance.
- Maintain running attendance records for every employee. The specific form of such records does not matter; it matters only that the supervisor is constantly aware of who is working, who has called in sick, and who has been out and when. Once organized to do so the supervisor may maintain such records manually without a great deal of difficulty. However, a growing number of organizations use computer systems that regularly provide supervisors with running attendance records of all personnel.
- Let the "pattern" absentees know that management is aware of the practices that appear to be emerging. Pattern absentees are of course those employees whose "sick" days fall into patterns such as days before or after scheduled days off, days of scheduled weekend work, days immediately preceding or following holidays, or days immediately following vacations. Quite often the simple knowledge that supervision recognizes the practice is sufficient to prompt pattern absentees to alter their behavior. In this sense, knowledge alone is prevention.
- Have employees who are coming off sick days report personally to supervision. Properly applied, this practice can send two messages to an employee: This supervisor cares about my availability as a producer and

my health as an individual; and this supervisor is actively monitoring absenteeism. Once again, knowledge is often prevention.

- Reward good attendance when possible. It is only reasonble for a supervisor to delegate potentially interesting and challenging tasks to employees who have demonstrated their dependability; this stands as a welcome form of recognition to many employees. Even if it is not possible to parcel out favored assignments to employees exhibiting regular attendance, the least that the supervisor can do in the way of reward is to recognize personally an employee's good attendance. A simple, "Thank you—it's nice to know I can count on you" can go a long way.

Communication

Implicit in most of the points made about the prevention of absenteeism is the need for thorough employee communication. All employees need and deserve to know that:

- They are expected to be at work when scheduled to work, unless prior arrangements have been made or unless absence is unavoidable or at least advisable and supervision is so notified according to policy.
- Absenteeism places a strain on co-workers and on the department as a whole, and it often incurs extra operating costs. Absenteeism is never to be taken for granted.
- Attendance records are maintained and are reviewed regularly. Attendance is considered in evaluating work performance, and one's attendance record can influence pay raises and consideration for promotion.
- Failure to maintain acceptable attendance can lead to disciplinary action under the organization's policies.

Applying the Limits

Most business organizations address absenteeism in two particular forms: excessive absenteeism and unexcused absenteeism. Since one of these kinds of absenteeism is far easier to define and identify than the other, they are usually dealt with separately.

Although guidelines describing excessive absenteeism can be created, excessive absenteeism is difficult to define precisely and even more difficult to monitor consistently for all employees. Generally, excessive absenteeism might be described as using sick time as fast as it is earned, the patterning of absences (before day off, after day off, and so on), or the apparent combination of these practices. With these rough guidelines some organizations have associated specific numbers of absences during specific periods of time.

For example, in one organization the threshold of excessive absenteeism is described as two or more days' absence in each of three consecutive months. Such guidelines ordinarily apply only to excused absences; that is, absences for which the employee has, according to policy, telephoned the proper person or office to give notice of the absence.

Unexcused absence is far easier to define and to deal with. One occurrence of unexcused absence is simply a single scheduled day during which the employee does not show up for work and does not call in according to policy. An occurrence of unexcused absence is cause for the supervisor to initiate the progressive disciplinary process. A typical progression of disciplinary action for continued unexcused absence might go as follows:

- First occurrence: an oral warning, in combination with one-on-one counseling concerning the importance of being at work as scheduled or at least providing notice of absence so that proper coverage can be arranged;
- Second occurrence: a written warning concerning unexcused absenteeism;
- Third occurrence: an additional written warning and perhaps a suspension (time off without pay), or, perhaps if the occurrences have been concentrated over a brief period of time and no effort toward correction has been demonstrated, termination;
- Fourth occurrence: termination.

Still easier to address from a policy point of view—although there is nothing constructive about the outcome—is the case of multiple consecutive unexcused absences. A common policy is one that calls for an employee's termination if the person fails to show up for work on three consecutive scheduled days and does not call in on any of those days. Simply referred to on occasion as "three-days-no-show-no-call," this set of circumstances often triggers a registered letter from the organization's personnel department advising the person of the termination. As unusual as this may seem to people who behave responsibly regarding their employment, an organization that employs, for example, 2,000 to 3,000 employees may experience a dozen or so such terminations in the course of a year. Indeed, an occasional person may "resign" by leaving at the end of a particular workday and, without ever telling anyone, simply never return.

Sense and Sensitivity

Teminations based on absenteeism, particularly those that stem from patterned absences and the use of sick time as fast as it is accrued, rest on shaky ground at best. Although common sense may suggest to the supervisor that the employee who is crowding the border of excessive absenteeism may rarely be sick at all and may be playing the system for time off, as long as the employee has followed the rules, primarily the rules concerned with calling in a notification of absence within the proper time, the supervisor has little choice but to accept the employee's word for the illness at face value. However, all employees who clearly go beyond policy limits and enter the realm of excessive absenteeism, the ones known to have chronic health problems as well as the suspected malingerers, must be dealt with consistently under the policy. Some people who have truly been frequently ill may lose their jobs, as will a number of people who have simply been playing the system. It may seem harsh to suggest that some people lose their jobs because of illness, but whether well or ill the employee who continually fails to show up for work is not fulfilling the basic employment agreement and is perhaps causing necessary work to go undone or creating extra expense required to pay replacements.

Because some regular sick time users are such as a result of genuine illness, it behooves the supervisor to provide all possible guidance to employees who seem to be establishing records of excessive absenteeism. In addition to thorough counseling regarding the policies of the organization and the necessity to be at work when scheduled, this guidance should include the invitation for an employee to visit the employee health office for information and advice. Also, it can be helpful to have persons who are shaping up as chronic absentees report to the employee health office to be cleared for work after every absence even of only a single day. This may well place the person with real health problems in a position to receive medical assistance more readily, and it will occasionally place a malingerer in a position of sufficient visibility that he or she may cut back on the unwarranted use of sick time.

As noted, it is not up to the supervisor to render a judgment concerning the medical legitimacy of an employee's absence, nor is it the supervisor's place to attempt to offer medical advice. However, taking every chronic absentee's stated reasons at face value, the supervisor can point the employee toward sources of medical advice and assistance and tell the employee about various options for leaves of absence and such.

SICK TIME INCENTIVE APPROACHES

In an effort to deal with increasing levels of absenteeism and associated costs, and also to address the problem of sick time abuse, some organizations have adopted incentive approaches intended to encourage employees to think twice before calling in sick when it is not justified. Such approaches theoretically place the employee in a position to be able to gain something by avoiding the use of sick time.

The problem being addressed by the incentive approaches was partly caused by the very organizations now wishing to correct that problem; when they established their sick time benefits in the first place, they inadvertently laid the groundwork for sick time abuse. There is good reason to suggest that the amount of sick time extended to each employee by an organization itself determines the level of at least part of the abuse. In short, if an amount of sick time is available, some of it will be used; if less sick time is available, a correspondingly smaller amount will be used. Consider an example: As part of an informal survey conducted during the preparation of this chapter, the sick time benefits and the sick time usage of two hospitals were compared. One hospital made available to its employees 12 sick days per year, with one day's sick time credited for each month of service. The other hospital granted its employees 5 sick days per year, credited to each employee on the employee's anniversary date. In the hospital that extended its employees 12 days per year the sick time use averaged 6.7 days per employee per year. In the institution granting its employees 5 days sick time per year, the average usage per employee per year was 3.2 days.

This is not to suggest that extending employees a greater amount of sick time is necessarily bad; a generous sick time allotment has served many employees well when such time has been needed. The practice also makes for good employee relations. However, if a generous sick time allotment is not accompanied by constant attention to absenteeism, a certain amount of abuse can find its way into the system. Without constant attention to absenteeism, a few employees can always be counted on to abuse the system. The fault, then, lies not in providing a generous amount of sick time but rather in failing to take steps to assure that sick time is used only for its intended purpose—income protection for brief periods of illness or injury.

This discussion is not intended to suggest that incentive approaches to the control of sick time are undesirable. However, all approaches will not work with the same degree of effectiveness in all organizations. The characteristics of an organization and the patterns of sick time use of all of its employees need to be studied before a method is selected and implemented.

In addition to a thorough analysis of sick time in the organization and a financial projection of the likely impact of an incentive approach, one critical decision is required in any organization contemplating an incentive approach, a decision concerning the nature of sick time itself as a benefit. If the decision is not made consciously, in advance, it is then made by default when such a system is installed. That is the decision to change sick time from an insurance-type benefit to a form of entitlement. Sick time began as, and in most organizations remains, an insurance-type benefit to be used only if needed. Once an incentive approach is implemented and some employees begin to realize tangible benefits from it, sick time is no longer a form of insurance. It is then an entitlement, and as an entitlement it is going to cost the organization some money out of pocket. In most instances, of course, it is hoped that the savings realized from reduced sick time usage are more than enough to offset the new costs of the entitlement. All elements of cost must be addressed, at least as reasonable estimates, in a pro forma financial analysis of any proposed system. The kinds of information taken into account would include, for example, the fact that some employees who are absent for a day or two at a time are not replaced for that period but rather that their work awaits their return and the only costs incurred are for the sick days themselves, and the fact that certain other employees must be replaced while absent so their absence incurs the cost of replacement help (agency temporaries and per diem employees) as well as the cost of the sick time itself.

There are also intangible factors to consider in assessing a sick time incentive approach. In some instances a plan may be deemed worthwhile even though it clearly costs more than it saves if it has considerable employee relations value and promotes the organization as a decent place to work.

In addition to the fundmental decision concerning the nature of the sick time benefit, implementation of an incentive approach requires that a particular philosophical hurdle be cleared as well. Under normal conditions of employment, employees are expected to be at work when scheduled and to use their sick time only when needed for genuine illness or injury, in other words, not to abuse the system. Since it is the persons who do not abuse the system who are the primary recipients of tangible rewards under an incentive approach, this puts the organization in a position of actively rewarding people for simply doing what they are expected to do anyway under normal terms of employment.

Occasionally valid concerns are also expressed about undesirable and perhaps harmful changes in some employees' attendance patterns under an incentive approach. Foremost among these concerns is the fear that to avoid losing out on an incentive pay-off, employees will work even when they are ill and should not be working. The problem was well expressed by the personnel director of a hospital that adopted the practice of giving a year-end bonus to employees achieving perfect attendance when he said, "Employee reaction has been good and our people really love the program. But when we get into November and December and winter colds set in or the flu bug strikes, we have people dragging themselves to work when they really belong home in bed. They just hate to miss out on that bonus."

Types of Sick Time Incentive Schemes

A survey undertaken for this chapter revealed a number of incentive approaches to the handling of sick time. With occasionally differing numbers and proportions involved, all of these schemes have seen active use in various organizations.

1) Include sick time and other potential paid-time-off along with vacation under the earned time concept. That is, such benefits as sick time, vacation, and personal days are accumulated in a single bank as earned. When a day is used, whether for illness, vacation, or personal business, it is deducted from the bank. Under this approach sick time is a clear entitlement of value equivalent to vacation.

2) Provide a cash bonus to an employee who accumulates some specific total hours of sick time in a bank, or provide this bonus for an employee who has used no sick time over a given period (usually one year).

3) Pay off accumulated sick time at the time of an employee's termination or retirement, either at full day-for-day value or at some lesser percentage of accumulated sick time. For example, upon termination or retirement two days' worth of sick time might be converted to the dollar value of one day's vacation time.

4) Extend sick leave eligibility to part-time employees. (In many organizations part-time employees receive no sick time or receive sick time on a pro rata basis.) This practice would provide many part-time employees with a way to protect their jobs with accrued sick time. By itself this policy is simply a way of attempting to reduce turnover among part-time employees; coupled with one of the incentive payout schemes it places part-time employees on the same footing as full-time employees with regard to their potential for benefiting financially by reducing sick time use.

5) Redesignate a given number of each year's available sick days as "personal days." Since personal days could be used for family illness, personal business, and other needs, such use could reduce the likelihood of an employee claiming illness when such is not the case. This increases the likelihood that more of the sick time actually taken would be for genuine illness. Again coupled with an incentive payout scheme, it would increase the likelihood of reduced sick time abuse because employees know they can use their personal days as required without touching their sick days and still remain eligible for the incentive award.

6) Treat the accrual of sick time as a graduated benefit based on years of service, allowing fewer days per year for employees with lesser service. Since on the average the majority of sick time abuse occurs among employees with

less service, this practice caps the potential amount of abuse from that group while assuring that employees with greater service will remain able to take advantage of whatever incentive happens to be in place.

7) Install a sick time buy-back plan under which employees who do not use sick time for some particular period can "sell" it back to the organization at some particular rate. One-third to one-half the regular rates of pay are fairly common buy-back factors; for example, in an organization with such a plan an employee with a large sick time bank may be permitted to trade in 20 days of sick time from the bank for 10 days of pay. Most plans require the employee to maintain a specific minimum sick time bank and also limit the number of days an employee can trade in each year.

8) In a plan much like the foregoing except that the conversion is to vacation time instead of money, require that the employee maintain a certain minimum bank of sick time above which he or she can convert additional accrued sick time into vacation at some specified rate. Most generous, of course, would be one sick day traded for one vacation day. Perhaps more appropriate, since both organization and individual would stand to gain, would be the practice of trading in two or three sick days for one vacation day.

9) Under a flexible benefits approach, value sick time as benefits credits which, instead of being held in reserve as sick time that might never be used, may be traded in to pay for other benefits. For example, perhaps an employee who is regularly attending school could use accrued benefits credits to convert to tuition assistance above the normal limits of a tuition assistance program. Or an employee might choose to apply benefits credits to pay for a particular form of insurance coverage such as supplemental life insurance.

A Final Precaution

In addition to assessing carefully the possible cost impact and the potential employee relations gains, before implementing a sick time incentive system, it is also necessary to consider the likely impact on future options available to the organization. Employees, especially those who stand to gain something, will always welcome the introduction of a new benefit. And such a move that results in an overall increase in employee compensation is indeed a new benefit. However, if a sick time incentive approach does not work—and usually this will emerge only after some time has elapsed and a number of cost reports have been developed and analyzed—there may be a temptation on the part of top management to alter, replace, or abandon the system. However, the process is not readily reversible. Once implemented, such a system is immediately seen by employees as belonging to them. The instant that top management moves to cut back or eliminate the program, employees react negatively as they would to the reduction of any part of compensation.

There will undoubtedly be some employee relations problems in an organization that has no sick time incentive plan; many people who do not abuse the system feel put upon because they see the chronic abusers enjoying the reward of extra time off. However, such problems may pale by comparison with those encountered on the elimination of something that most employees have come to regard as an entitlement. Thus once in place, a sick time incentive system may, for better or worse, be permanent.

NOTES

1. Ronald J. Bula, "Absentee Control," *Personnel Journal* 63, no. 6 (June 1984): 56–60.
2. Ellis D. Roberts, *Absenteeism Hurts* (Timonium, Md.: Kirkley Press, 1969), p. 5.
3. Bula, "Absenteeism Control," pp. 56–60.
4. Governor's Office of Employee Relations, *Supervisor's Guide to Administering Sick Leave Policies* (Albany: State of New York, 1982), p. 11.

Chapter 12

Workers' Compensation, Unemployment, and Disability

No gain is so certain as that which proceeds from the economical use of what you already have.

Latin Proverb

Chapter Objectives

- Establish the importance of workers' compensation, unemployment, and disability as cost elements of sometimes significant impact on the organization.
- Identify the role of the supervisor in attempting to control these elements of cost.
- Explore the supervisor's possible opportunities for productively utilizing employees who may be returned to work from workers' compensation or disability at only partial capacity.

Workers' compensation, unemployment compensation, and disability are often easy to ignore or to forget entirely. Most of the ability to control the costs of workers' compensation, unemployment compensation, and disability appears to lie beyond the responsibility of the individual supervisor, usually residing in some branch of the human resource activity or perhaps with a more specialized risk management function. Regardless of apparent limitations on the opportunity for direct control, however, the supervisor can nevertheless exert a certain degree of influence over some aspects of these elements of cost.

The cost elements receiving primary attention in this chapter are more thoroughly defined as follows:

- Workers' compensation is compensation for costs arising from injury or illness that is directly related to an individual's employment. It covers medical expenses arising from such injury or illness, and it compensates for a portion of wages lost because of that injury or illness.
- Unemployment compensation is compensation for a portion of the wages lost because of periods of unemployment that are beyond the control of the individual.
- Disability, often referred to as short-term disability or simply DBL, is insurance coverage that provides compensation for a portion of the wages lost because of injury or illness that is not related to one's employment.

Workers' compensation, unemployment, and disability often receive scant attention because they are thought of by many people, employees and supervisors alike, simply as forms of insurance—we pay our premiums and occasionally someone collects. However, there are a number of different forms of insurance and there are different ways of determining an organization's premium. Regarding these particular forms of insurance coverage an organization is ordinarily, to use insurance language, "experience rated." This means that the premium paid by the organization is based directly on that organization's claims experience. In short, under experience rating when the claims increase, the premiums increase accordingly. Thus workers' compensation, unemployment, and disability require conscientious control as do all other costs of doing business.

WORKERS' COMPENSATION

Workers' compensation laws are in effect in all 50 states as well as in American Samoa, the District of Columbia, Guam, Puerto Rico, and the Virgin Islands.

According to estimates released by the Social Security Administration, workers' compensation costs paid out nationwide on behalf of employees during 1972 amounted to $4 billion. During 1981 these same costs amounted to $15 billion, representing an increase of 270 percent of workers' compensation costs in just ten calendar years. Individual states experienced widely varying workers' compensation cost increases, ranging from a low of 114 percent for New York to a high of 883 percent for Maine.[1]

The medical benefits paid under workers' compensation laws generally amount to full actual medical expenses. The amount of benefit paid for compensation for lost wages varies considerably from state to state, but nationwide the most common benefit paid amounts to two-thirds of wages up to some specified maximum. Most states place limits on both maximum and minimum weekly benefits, the total number of weeks that benefits can be received, and the total dollar amount of benefit eligibility. Most states also provide lifetime payment for permanent disability, and some states also pay additional amounts for dependents, rehabilitation services, and other benefits.[2]

For some time a number of study groups have been active in several states, seeking ways to increase workers' benefits while lowering employers' costs.[3] During 1983, in the United States more than 1,100 proposals affecting workers' compensation benefits and payment were introduced in various legislatures and 232 of these proposals were signed into law. Most of these legislative actions increased workers' compensation costs to employers, some significantly.[4]

Workers' Compensation Costs and the Supervisor

As already suggested, much of the ability to control workers' compensation costs may lie beyond the supervisor. The supervisor is but one of a number of people in the organization who have separate but none too distinctly defined roles in controlling workers' compensation costs.

By far the best approach to the control of workers' compensation costs involves the operation of an effective accident prevention program. Here the supervisor's role is one of remaining constantly aware of the requirements of the program and assuring that all requirements are thoroughly observed by all employees. The supervisor must assure that employees:

- are thoroughly educated in safe work practices, including, in the health care setting, safe lifting techniques and safe handling of needles and other pointed implements (since puncture wounds, as well as back strains resulting from improper lifting, are among the most common on-the-job injuries experienced by health care workers);

- adhere to all of the safety rules in place in the organization, those rules mandated by arms of government and particular insurance carriers as well as safety rules established by the institution;
- make full, appropriate use of all required safety equipment in the performance of their jobs.

In pursuing an effective accident prevention program, it is clearly the responsibility of the supervisor to maintain a high level of consciousness of the need for safety among employees. In doing so it may be necessary for the supervisor to deal directly with the unsafe practices of employees in a disciplinary way. A violation of a safety rule is as much of a transgression as a violation of any other work rule or policy. Violators must be counseled appropriately, and if they continue to be violators they must eventually be dealt with through the progressive disciplinary process.

Another important, if somewhat indirect, way of approaching the control of workers' compensation costs is through the organization's pre-employment physical examination. Although the organization cannot refuse to hire an individual who may exhibit a "qualifying handicap" under the anti-discrimination laws, there is nevertheless considerable flexibility available for determining whether a potential new employee carries a high risk of becoming a workers' compensation case. The institution is within its rights to determine whether a prospective employee has a pre-existing medical condition that could be aggravated by the job and could thus cause health problems for the employee as well as increase the organization's exposure to workers' compensation costs. In many organizations the supervisor is protected by a firm policy that requires every new employee to receive medical clearance before starting work. However, in an organization in which practices might be less well organized, it would be in the best interest of the supervisor to resist agreeing to start a new employee on the job until after medical clearance has been obtained.

The supervisor should also be part of the process of closely monitoring workers' compensation claims and challenging those that appear to be inappropriate. To monitor claims properly it is necessary that the supervisor be thorough and timely in providing all documentation that may have a bearing on a claim, that is, all necessary incident reports and accident reports should be provided as soon as possible after the fact and should be clear and detailed.

There will often be a question of whether a particular injury did or did not occur during working time or on the institution's property, and it may be necessary to take steps to determine whether workers' compensation is appropriate (an on-the-job occurrence) or whether the case more appropriately falls under short-term disability (an off-the-job occurrence). Employees will occasionally report off-the-job accidents as occurring on the job, especially in those states and work organizations where the weekly workers' compensation benefit exceeds the short-term disability benefit or where a short-term disability benefit does not exist. After an injured employee's personal physician, the employee's supervisor is often the next most important person in determining whether a given occurrence does or does not fall under workers' compensation.

UNEMPLOYMENT COMPENSATION

The Social Security Act of 1935 made the individual states responsible for their own unemployment compensation insurance programs. A federal tax was imposed on employers, but most of this tax could be offset by state taxes. All programs were to be controlled at the state level.

Unemployment compensation insurance programs are in effect in all states and in the District of Columbia and Puerto Rico. Unemployment compensation is an area of active change throughout the states. During 1983, 43 states plus the District of Columbia legislated changes in their unemployment compensation insurance laws. Most of these changes resulted in increased benefits to employees and increased costs to the employer.[5]

Although differences exist throughout the country, employers are generally subject to experience rating, that is, employers are taxed according to their past records; thus an employer which decreases its unemployment will also decrease its unemployment tax bill. The majority of business organizations—virtually all profit-making businesses—are taxed directly using experience-based rates established by the various states. However, in a number of states nonprofit organizations, including most health care institutions, pay for their unemployment on direct experience rather than paying a tax based on a percentage of payroll, that is, such organizations pay their unemployment costs on a dollar-for-dollar basis, paying actual costs as they are incurred.

Since unemployment compensation is intended to make up for wages lost due to periods of unemployment beyond the employee's control, unemployment compensation is ordinarily not made available to people who voluntarily resign their employment or who are discharged for cause. Rather, unemployment compensation is intended primarily for employees who are laid off through no fault of their own or who otherwise find that their services are no longer required. Also generally qualifying for unemployment compensation are individuals who have been dismissed due to the apparent inability to meet the requirements of their positions. In this regard an employee's failure on the grounds of performance is not treated as harshly as out-and-out misconduct that might result in discharge for cause. Also, in a relatively few states employees who are on strike can receive unemployment compensation after a specified waiting period (six or more weeks from the start of the strike).

The Supervisor's Role in Unemployment Cost Control

To the extent that it is possible for the supervisor to regulate or moderate certain kinds of employee turnover, it is possible for the supervisor to have an effect on the institution's unemployment costs. Following are some general guidelines for the supervisor to consider:

1) The exercise of care and thoroughness in hiring will help to reduce the chances of acquiring an employee who may turn out to be unable to do the job. It must be acknowledged that it is not possible to refine the hiring process to the point where one always knows that the right choice is being made, but nevertheless if the supervisor sticks to normal minimum education and experience requirements and does not rush to a decision based on insufficient information or an insufficient number of candidates, it is often possible to head off performance problems before they can begin. And in the process of heading off potential performance problems the supervisor will also be avoiding potential unemployment costs.

2) Regarding hiring, orientation, and especially the application of disciplinary action, the supervisor should scrupulously follow all of the policies of the organization and all essential legal processes. Disciplinary actions, especially those in a series of such actions that may eventually result in termination, are especially important. All such actions need to be thoroughly documented and should be taken strictly in accordance with the organization's policies and Equal Employment Opportunity (EEO) guidelines. Since many nonlegitimate claims for unemployment compensation are entered, it is frequently necessary to use records of disciplinary actions to refute such claims. Also, since the acknowledged primary purpose of much disciplinary action is the correction of employee behavior, it is frequently necessary to produce documentation of a series of related actions to demonstrate that an employee had been given the opportunity to correct the errant behavior but failed to do so.

3) Regarding the inability of an employee to meet the requirements of a job, if it is at all possible the supervisor should act to remove a substandard employee during the organization's probationary period. It must be recognized that often the organization's probationary period is too short a time in which to be able to make a definite decision concerning an employee's ability, especially the ability of an apparently marginal employee. However, the probationary period is often sufficient to give the supervisor a strong indication of where the new employee is heading. Separation for performance-related reasons is usually easier to justify outside of the organization if it occurs by the expiration of an understood probationary period. Also, because

an institution's unemployment costs are related to the length of time an employee has worked for that organization, separation by the end of the probationary period reduces the organization's cost exposure.

4) Working in conjunction with the organization's personnel department, the supervisor should challenge all unemployment claims that appear inappropriate. Many people automatically file for unemployment compensation regardless of why or how they left their positions; they have nothing to lose by trying. Many will state their reasons for termination clearly in their favor, and it then becomes necessary for the organization to dispute such claims to avoid unemployment costs. If a claim goes undisputed by the organization, the employee, deserving or not, will automatically collect unemployment compensation. Thus every effort should be made to dispute each inappropriate claim.

5) The supervisor should consider the use of temporary help in the department when it is known that certain requirements are only of short duration. There may often be the temptation to hire a person to cover a given need and terminate the individual when the need has passed; however, this automatically places the organization in a position of exposure to unemployment costs. On the other hand, the use of temporary help, engaged specifically for certain tasks or for known brief periods of time, will avoid such costs. In most parts of the country it requires six months (26 weeks) of work for a single employer to move the organization to the point of maximum exposure to unemployment cost, so any particular need of less than six months that can be covered by temporary help eliminates the organization's exposure to unemployment costs.

DISABILITY

Unlike workers' compensation and unemployment compensation, which are statutory requirements throughout the entire country, short-term DBL is not a widespread legal requirement. However, whether coverage is in place by virtue of the employer's choice rather than by requirement of law, it nevertheless requires the same level of conscientious attention to the control of associated costs.

As of the middle of 1983, nonoccupational disability laws were in effect in only five states (California, Hawaii, New Jersey, New York, and Rhode Island) and Puerto Rico. All of these legislated disability plans cover employers of one or more employees. All except Rhode Island permit private plans to be used in place of the state plan as long as the private plan is equal to or better than the state plan (the lone exception is Rhode Island which permits no private plans except as supplements to the required state plan).

The length of time that disability extends and the amount of benefits paid have been increasing steadily for several years. In 1977, 62.9 percent of all employees in the country were covered under disability plans providing up to 26 weeks of benefits. By the end of 1982 this figure had grown to 76 percent.[6] In 1977, 32.9 percent of employees in the country were covered by plans that cut off all benefits at 13 weeks. By the end of 1982, only 19.7 percent had benefits terminated at 13 weeks.[7]

During 1982, 24.3 percent of employees in the country were covered by short-term disability plans that paid up to a maximum benefit of $250 per week. However, a number of plans were, and still are, paying benefits as low as $60 per week.[8]

As with the other forms of coverage discussed in this chapter, an organization is usually experience rated regarding disability. Any year's actual experience, that is, claims actually paid, is directly reflected in next year's premium rates. Therefore, most organizations pay dollar for dollar; they eventually pay the total actual costs of all claims, plus administrative expenses.

Control of Disability Costs

From the point of view of the individual supervisor, the control of disability costs is extremely difficult. That action which has the greatest impact on the organization's disability costs as a whole is usually that which is undertaken by the whole organization—for example, self-insurance, administration of one's own claims, general employee health and safety programs, and clear, organization-wide disability procedures with precise responsibilities identified. The individual supervisor can:

- provide employees with information that the organization may supply concerning personal health and safety in general, and information on certain hazards or illnesses in particular;
- urge employees to take advantage of the annual physical examinations or health assessments that many organizations offer, and also always be prepared to refer employees to the organization's employee health office when questions arise or problems become apparent;
- scrupulously fulfill all departmental responsibilities in following disability procedures, assuring that all necessary forms are thoroughly executed in a timely fashion.

FURTHER OPPORTUNITIES FOR SUPERVISORY CONTROL

The supervisor who occasionally has employees absent on workers' compensation or short-term disability—and surely this applies to all supervisors at one time or another—will occasionally have related opportunities to help control costs. This section examines some of the alternatives that are occasionally available to the supervisor.

"Light Duty Only"

Many employees who are out on workers' compensation or disability are first cleared to return to work on "light duty only." However, if such light duty is not available the compensation or DBL may continue. Also, an occasional employee may receive medical clearance to return on a part-time basis only. However, there are often problems in coming up with the light-duty or part-time assignment for an employee who is not yet ready to return to his or her regular duties. There may be a limited number of exclusively light-duty positions in the facility, and it may seem as easy to allow an individual to continue on compensation or DBL until that person receives medical clearance to return to his or her original position. However, there are costs, often unnecessary costs, associated with the continuation of compensation or DBL.

Consider, for example, an employee who goes off on DBL under a system that pays up to six months' benefits. Assume too that this employee could return on the basis of "light duty only" after only two months of absence. If this occurs in a state in which the average disability benefit is $135 per week, and if light duty is not made available, this employee could conceivably remain out of work, collecting $135 per week, for an additional four months before benefits ran out or full job duties could be resumed.

It is conceded, however, that it could be extremely difficult to justify light duty, for example, for:

- a maintenance worker who finds it medically necessary to remain off his feet for ten weeks;
- a nurse who cannot be permitted to lift more than 25 pounds at a time for a month;
- a transportation aide who is restricted from pushing a loaded cart for three months.

But all such persons may be collecting workers' compensation or DBL when they are not working, and the full cost of those benefits paid goes directly back to the organization.

It is occasionally possible to save money if an employee can be put to work doing something that someone else would have to be paid for doing. Consider, for example, a maintenance worker who ordinarily makes $7.50 per hour ($300 per week) who is out of work and collecting $135 per week on disability. Assume that this maintenance worker, who has been cleared to return to "light duty only," is used to fill temporarily the position of a maintenance clerk who would ordinarily earn $6.00 per hour ($240 per week). The maintenance worker would of course be paid his normal pay, so the organization would be paying $60 extra per week to maintain an employee in the clerical position. However, overall the organization would be saving $75 per week ($135 for DBL, less the $60 pay in excess wges) to cover the clerical position. Thus it would make sense to cover temporary requirements or at least to temporarily fill open positions of a light-duty nature with individuals who would otherwise be drawing compensation or DBL payments.

The areas or circumstances that should be examined closely for light duty possibilities in a health care institution include the following:

- A clinic or outpatient area may offer some limited opportunity for light duty assignments because the majority of outpatients are mobile and do not require constant bending and lifting by staff. Such an area might provide a temporary assignment for the nurse who is recovering from back strain.

- Desk-bound clerical work may be appropriate for light duty assignment when available. As in the example of the maintenance man who could not perform his regular duties for a particular period of time, the organization may pay more money to get the work done but will be able to avoid more than an offsetting amount of workers' compensation or disability costs. It is also possible that such an assignment could avoid the use of a temporary employee to cover a particular clerical need, or the assignment itself may perhaps be made available by forestalling the hiring of a full-time clerical employee until after the maintenance worker is back on his regular job. Even in the absence of a particular full-time opening, either permanent or temporary, a light duty employee may perhaps be productively used to cover for vacations or illness again without the need for resorting to outside temporary help.

- A light duty employee can occasionally be put to good use in orienting or training new employees. Knowledgeable employees with temporary physical limitations may be able to teach specific skills and processes to others; for example, the nurse on light duty because of physical limitations may be used to train new nursing assistants or to orient newly hired nurses in particular nursing specialty areas.

- Knowledgeable employees restricted to light duty can sometimes be used for inventorying equipment or supplies. For example, a nurse with lifting restrictions could inventory all nursing-unit stock areas; a maintenance worker who temporarily cannot cope with the normal physical strain of the job could be used to identify and tag all stored equipment.

- A knowledgeable employee limited to light duty can often be productively used in reviewing and updating job descriptions for a department. Such a person might also be gainfully employed in auditing the status of policies and procedures and recommending changes to bring them up to date.

In implementing some of the foregoing suggestions, it is essential to consider the status of the cost center's personnel budget. If the department is running well within budget, that is, less has been spent for the year to date for personnel than was allocated, it is occasionally appropriate to consider bringing in a light duty employee. Although a pure "make-work" assignment is never considered appropriate from a financial point of view, it often may seem to make sense from an employee relations perspective. None of this is intended to suggest seriously that "busy work" be invented simply to keep an employee on the payroll; while perhaps appearing as the humane thing to do, this invariably makes poor business sense in today's health care operating environment. Rather, the suggested light duty assignments should represent work that, although presently not pressing or of any particular priority, must eventually be done by someone. If the supervisor can stay within the cost center's personnel budget while making use of light duty employees, some costs of workers' compensation or disability can be avoided and the organization's employee relations can often be enhanced.

As a general rule, if an employee who has been cleared to return on light duty only can be used in a less-than-usual capacity and this can be done within the limits of the approved budget, and this person does some form of necessary work, it is to the economic advantage of the department and the organization to do so. Of course, if the department is running over the limits of its personnel budget, anything that might remotely appear to be "make-work"—such as a task of low priority, one which will eventually have to be done but for which no sense of urgency or necessity has yet developed— will likely be regarded in just that light. However, the use of an employee in less than the person's usual capacity can often be justified if the work is considered necessary and if the use of the person will avoid the employment of temporary help or forestall the hiring of another permanent employee.

Outside Agencies

In many states there are government and social agencies that specialize in guiding the career reorientation of workers who, because of the permanent effects of illness or injury, can no longer do the same kinds of work they had been doing. For example, New York has its Office of Vocational

Rehabilitation (OVR), and a number of other states have equivalent services. These agencies can often be called upon, at no cost to the organization, to perform complete aptitude testing for an employee who is faced with learning how to live and work with new physical or medical limitations following an injury or illness. Such testing frequently provides clues as to the directions that might be taken in looking for placement possibilities for the worker with permanent limitatons. Further, some of these agencies provide some level of funding for periods of on-the-job training for employees who are channeled into different lines of work because of their limitations.

The existence of such agencies and the extent of their involvement in rehabilitating workers vary considerably from state to state, so one can only generalize regarding this avenue of approach for the organization. However, one's starting point for acquiring specific information may lie as close as the nearest metropolitan telephone directory under the listings for state, city, or county agencies.

HIDDEN COSTS

By and large the costs of workers' compensation, unemployment, and DBL remain hidden to the individual supervisor. However, to call a given cost element a hidden cost is really to say only that it is hidden to some people, not all. Even the most well-hidden of all hidden costs will be visible—perhaps distressingly so—to the person who has to pay the bills or balance the books. The individual supervisor can play a valuable role in the control of such costs by:

- first, finding out who in the organization, by name and title, is primarily responsible for administering and monitoring workers' compensation, unemployment, and disability;
- asking these responsible people for department-specific cost information —on a case-by-case basis, the department's share of workers' compensation, unemployment, and disability costs;
- completely fulfilling all supervisory responsibilities in the timely processing of appropriate forms and the thorough, timely provision of incident and accident reports, and the thorough, timely documentation of disciplinary processes when they are involved;
- reaching out to those persons with organization responsibility for workers' compensation, unemployment, and disability, and becoming involved in active efforts to control such costs.

NOTES

1. "Cost of Work Comp Benefits up 270% in 10 Years: Study," *Business Insurance*, March 19, 1982, p. 6.
2. "Workers' Compensation Laws: Income Benefits for Total Disabilities—January 1984," *Bulletin to Management*, June 14, 1984, pp. 4-6.
3. "States Betting on Variety of Work Comp Reforms," *Business Insurance*, February 27, 1984, p. 1.
4. LaVerne C. Tinsley, "Workers' Compensation: Significant Enactments in 1983," *Monthly Labor Review*, February 1984, pp. 55-61.
5. Diana Runner, "Changes in Unemployment Insurance Legislation during 1983," *Monthly Labor Review*, February 1984, pp. 46-54.
6. "Disability Plans Becoming More Generous, Survey Says," *Business Insurance*, January 24, 1983, p. 13.
7. Ibid.
8. Ibid.

Part V

Other Resources: Walls, Equipment, and Everything Else That Money Can Buy

Chapter 13

Controlling Nonwage Costs

There can be no economy when there is no efficiency.

Lord Beaconsfield

Chapter Objectives

- Place a department's nonwage costs into perspective as a frequently minor cost category (when compared with personnel costs) but nevertheless a critical consideration in budgetary control.
- Present guidelines for the supervisor to consider in attempting to control the costs of office supplies, photocopying, telephone use, and other important elements of nonwage cost associated with the operation of a department.

Although percentages are bound to vary from one organization to another, in the average health care organization, and specifically in the average hospital, total personnel costs, including benefits as well as direct wages and salaries, fall in the range of 55 to 60 percent of total operating costs. The other 40 to 45 percent is made up of nonwage costs.[1]

Realistically, a considerable proportion of an organization's nonwage cost goes for expenditures that lie beyond the control of the individual supervisor. Such expenditures ordinarily include interest and debt reduction payments, various insurance premiums, capital expenditures made on behalf of the organization as a whole, and fees paid for a variety of services that may not relate to the individual supervisor in any way. Certainly most supervisors need not be concerned with loan amortization and interest payments and many other expenditures beyond his or her control. However, when all such expenditures are taken into consideration there nevertheless remains some level of nonwage expenditure that rightly is the responsibility of the individual supervisor.

The amount of nonwage cost for which the supervisor is responsible will vary greatly according to the department or function of concern. Functional areas that are large scale users of purchased supplies, areas, for example, like clinical laboratories, can experience nonwage costs in the range of 30 to 40 percent of their departmental budgets. For an individual department, 40 percent is fairly representative of the high end of the range of the nonwage costs. In a nursing department it is not unusual for the proportion of nonwage cost to fall in the range of 15 to 20 percent of the budget.

Near the low end of the scale are the nonmedical, office-based support functions in which nonwage costs frequently fall in the range of four to seven percent of budget. Common functions found in this category are accounting, personnel, and other such support activities. Therefore, at an absolute minimum the individual supervisor will have nonwage cost responsibilities that amount to at least four or five percent of the department's budget.

One's initial reaction to the foregoing might be to wonder why one should be much concerned with a mere four or five percent of the budget. Although the organization's total cost may amount to 60 percent for personnel and 40 percent for nonwage items, the individual department's budget may be allocated 96 percent to personnel and only four percent to nonwage items. It is correct to suggest that much more of the supervisor's time and attention is legitimately focused on controlling personnel costs. However, it often requires only a small swing in a department's operating results, perhaps even considerably less than one percent of budget to make a difference between positive or negative bottom-line results for the entire department. There are at least two clear reasons for suggesting that the supervisor has a genuine need to monitor nonwage costs:

- The supervisor is directly answerable to his or her immediate superior for performance against budget.
- The entire organization's budget performance is no more than the sum of the budget performances of all individual supervisors and managers.

For the individual cost center supervisor whose primary concern is getting work done through the efforts of a group of people, nonwage costs may include all or most of the following: employee education and training; office supplies (pens and paper and forms and all else that go to support day-to-day activities); photocopying and other reproduction services; dues to organizations and subscriptions to publications and information services; books, and possibly films and audio and video tapes; miscellaneous food expenditures; and maintenance and repairs for typewriters, calculators, computer terminals, and other office equipment.

Also pertinent to the department—often budgeted for the institution as a whole, but ultimately controllable within each department—are the costs associated with telephone service and the cost of postage.

An individual department's nonwage cost may also include purchased services such as temporary clerical or technical help secured through agencies. This certainly involves personnel but since the organization does not enter into a formal employment relationship with these persons it is a common practice to reflect the projected cost of such expenditures on the nonwage side of the budget.

As suggested earlier, most of a supervisor's control effort will be focused on the cost and productivity of personnel. In dealing with nonwage costs it would hardly be productive, and might well be counterproductive, for the supervisor to establish elaborate, costly, and time-consuming controls. Thus it is suggested that the supervisor monitor most nonwage costs through the use of simple common sense controls and through the use of knowledge and visibility within the work group. Specifically:

- knowledge of the employees in the group as to the cost and value of the nonwage items at their disposal;
- visibility of the supervisor's awareness, interest, and active involvement in controlling such costs.

The following sections offer suggestions for monitoring the nonwage expenditures that fall fully or at least partially under the control of the individual supervisor.

SUPPLIES

This discussion primarily concerns office supplies. It does not specifically include the control of pharmaceuticals, although medical supplies that are not subject to legal control requirements should be subject to common sense rules of supply control. Also, many pharmaceuticals, especially controlled substances, are subject to such a variety of legal requirements that they are in effect already controlled if all applicable regulations are observed.

Inventory Control for the Supervisor

Every department has an interest in inventory control, although perhaps not to the extent of a materiel management department or a central supply department that must maintain a high-dollar-value stock for the entire organization. Materiel management or central supply managers apply sophisticated inventory control processes, including the use of economic-order-point formulas. While desirable in such settings, such approaches are not for the individual supervisor; applying these in most departments would cause expenditure of excess amounts of time and money in controlling small items and limited expenditures. Rather, a common sense approach to ordering, storing, and dispensing supplies is in order. The supervisor should try to keep everything that is needed readily available without tying up excess amounts of money and precious space with excess stock. Following are some guidelines for the supervisor to consider:

1) *Assign specific responsibility.* One person, preferably someone who is there most of the time, should be aware of what is available in the department, where it is kept, and the status of any outstanding orders. Ideally, one additional person should be sufficiently knowledgeable as to be able to fill in when the primary assigned individual is not available. Thus there should be specific, assigned responsibility in the department for ordering, stocking, and perhaps even releasing supplies. This function might best be performed by the office manager, if there is one, or by the department secretary, perhaps with the department supervisor functioning as backup when necessary.

It is advisable to keep all of the department's stock in one central location if possible, preferably near the responsible person but also accessible to the employees in the department if they serve themselves. It is also helpful to provide a need list on the door of the supply cabinet or in some other prominent place so people can note what they need that is not ordinarily stocked or that may be in short supply.

2) *Develop rules of thumb.* If a number of high-dollar items or many, many smaller items adding up to big money are stocked, one is in the inventory business and must use formal control systems. However, most supervisors need only informal rules to attempt to achieve the best mix of the cost of:

- obtaining stock;
- holding stock (the dollars tied up in stock and the space occupied);
- ordering stock and monitoring usage.

It is suggested that the supervisor develop simple rules based on experience, perhaps on the order of: "For item No. XX, order four dozen whenever the quantity on hand (plus the quantity on order, if it is an outside purchase) falls below 18. Review weekly."

Regarding this sample rule one might know, for example, that four dozen of the item will last at least three months and that on the average about 12 are used between the time an order is placed and the time an order arrives. The extra six (18 minus 12), strictly a judgment call, represent a margin of safety should it take longer than usual to obtain the item.

For an item that is always acquired from an inside source, the guideline might appear as follows: On the regular weekly order, request three packs of yellow pads when the last pack in the cabinet has been opened.

3) *Make employees conscious of waste and its cost.* Waste often exists and is often encouraged because there seems to be an endless supply of all items. Employees sometimes do not worry about what they use, and how much, when they know they can obtain more quite easily. Lack of consciousness about waste and its cost is manifested as lack of concern. A person who works in an office, for example, may seldom think about the cost of standard yellow tablets. But in one organization when a system error caused the materiel management department to run completely out of yellow tablets, departments that had also run out were forced to look for what they could find. Said one supervisor, "I know I occasionally put away partial tablets in various files or left them with my working notes here and there. So I asked everybody in the department to make a pass through their stuff and look for yellow pads, and I did the same. We came up with enough partial tablets out of desks and filing cabinets to hold us for nearly a month."

For the sake of employee cost consciousness, one institution maintains an inventory list on the door of every supply cabinet. In addition to indicating the reorder points for all significant items, this list shows the dollar cost of each item in stock. Anyone who looks at such a list to determine if a desired item is in the cabinet will also see the cost of that item. Such practices create an awareness of cost.

4) *Perform a periodic physical inventory.* The supervisor, as well as the individual designated as responsible for supplies, should learn exactly what is available and should develop a sense for what is or is not in actual use. This information should be used to update the department's informal order rules. Also, a periodic physical inventory is extremely helpful in encouraging one to straighten up the contents of supply storage cabinets.

5) *Monitor turnover.* A simple indicator of turnover per unit of time may be determined by dividing the cost of supplies consumed during a time period by the average dollar value of supplies in inventory and expressing the results as a percent. For example, 50 percent turnover in a period of three months indicates that half the dollar value of the total stock has been used and replaced during that time. One can manipulate turnover by changing the department's rule of thumb—specifically, by reducing quantities ordered and reducing the specific quantities that trigger ordering. Generally, the higher one can move the turnover rate without running out of supplies, the better off the department will be. A higher rate of turnover means that less money is tied up in idle stock at any time and less space is consumed for storing supplies.

6) *Periodically clean out obsolete supplies.* The department should periodically dispose of surplus or obsolete inventory. Though some may have monetary value, as long as it has no present or foreseeable value to the department it is no more than clutter that takes up space and perhaps also adds to the difficulty experienced in finding things. However, a great deal of material that should simply be discarded is retained for long periods simply because people are afraid to throw things away. They are often hesitant to discard anything that is of obvious value, and they frequently take refuge in the possibility that "we may need it someday."

Occasionally some items of excess inventory are salvageable for cash. For example, costly notebook binders, the covers of which have been printed for specific uses that no longer apply, can often be salvaged through a process that removes the printing. If such is possible the organizaton's purchasing department can usually arrange to dispose of the binders for their salvage value. Also, stocks of ribbon and paper tapes for office machines that are no longer used in the department can often be disposed of, again through the purchasing department, at some value, or can often be redirected toward departments that still use the appropriate machines and can thus use these supplies. However, if all reasonable possibilities have been exhausted and items of supposed value cannot be salvaged for other use, nothing remains except to discard them. Past cost notwithstanding, an item's true value is determined by its usefulness, and if it has no present or foreseeable usefulness, it has no value.

The true causes of an unfavorable variance in a department's use of supplies could include any of the following:

- waste occurring during use by employees;
- theft or pilferage;
- higher quality or more expensive products ordered and used than are truly required;
- introduction of new procedures that render present supplies obsolete;
- changes in specifications in products used, rendering present supplies obsolete;
- product substitutions, in which higher priced alternatives are used;
- loss occurring during storing or handling.

Within most departments, a simple awareness of the cost of supplies, plus common sense monitoring of usage, should be sufficient. The individual supervisor need not "count paper clips" in order to maintain reasonable control over supply usage. One should put the emphasis where the dollars are. That is, the supervisor might reasonably want to "count" telephone handsets or calculators or even staplers or leather gloves or the like, but for smaller items used in the normal conduct of business the foregoing guidelines should suffice.

COPYING

Today's photocopiers will do so much work so well and so rapidly and are relied upon so heavily that one wonders how we ever got along without them in the world of business. Consider as an example the manuscript of any book that you might now happen to be reading. A book manuscript is often produced in triplicate, with the original and one copy going to the publisher and one copy being retained by the author. The necessary two copies 30 to 35 years ago would have been created by using two sheets of carbon paper and painstakingly making every necessary correction on both copies as well as on the original. But even with a copy on hand to back up the original, the publisher's processes would have been much different and much less efficient than they are today. Often a book manuscript will go through several reviewers. With inexpensive, rapidly produced photocopies available, today's reviewers ordinarily see the book in parallel with each other; years ago this and other activities had to take place serially because each person involved had to work on the same copy. There is no doubt that photocopying has dramatically changed the procedures applied in running most business enterprises.

However, there is also little doubt that the rapidly advancing technology of photocopying has spawned much of its own increase in demand. The faster and cheaper photocopying has become, the more copies we have generated and the less careful we have been about wasting copies.

Probably the majority of copy machines in the average health care organizaton are shared. Outside of a very few heavily paper-oriented departments, not many departments can justify the use of a dedicated machine. Of course some dedicated machines may be placed primarily for the sake of convenience, and this may make sense if, for example, long walking distances and regular waiting times are involved in the use of the nearest available machine. Considering staff time, stat copying, and the volume of work that must be copied, a dedicated copier for a specific department may well be justified. Also, dedicated copiers for certain departments such as medical records or personnel may be justified by the need for confidentiality as well as by volume.

For economic considerations, or perhaps as a matter of policy, some machines may be owned outright by the organization. In such circumstances the organization buys all of the supplies and either performs service and maintenance internally or buys them from outside. But while a growing number of copy machines are owned outright by various organizations, many machines continue to be leased from copy machine companies. A variety of leasing arrangements are available, including the common one of paying a flat charge per month which includes a prespecified number of copies above which a nominal amount is paid for each additional copy. However, whether a given machine is owned outright or leased, every copy that is produced represents a cost to the department.

A major problem of copy machine use that has been around as long as the machines themselves is personal copying. Few organizations will probably ever stamp out personal copying completely, except perhaps by applying means that are far more costly than the cost of the unwarranted copies (and means that are also highly distasteful to employees and supervisors alike). Various approaches to the rigid control of copy machines have been attempted from time to time. For example:

- One relatively small hospital operated by a religious order owned one copy machine. No one was allowed to do any copying except a single, elderly nun who was assigned full time to run the machine and do all of the organization's copying.
- Another relatively small hospital attempted to staff its sole copy machine with one volunteer at all times during the normal business day. However, it turned out to be practically impossible to retain a reliable volunteer presence at all times so the practice was abandoned.

• Some organizations have employed full-time copy clerks to operate centralized machines. This practice has proven economical only in centralized duplicating departments in large organizations.

Among practices that supervision and higher management can consider for reasonable control of copying are:

1) *Locate machines where they are highly visible.* When copy machines are located in highly visible, open areas—as opposed to being located in out-of-the-way corners, stock rooms, closets, and such—employees are less likely to run a large volume of personal material. In visible, open settings, people are more aware that the material they are copying will be visible to passersby, people working in the area, and people waiting in line for the machine.

2) *Post copying limitations clearly at every machine.* A clearly posted prohibition against copying personal material is not going to stop the determined individual from copying personal material. However, should the supervisor eventually find it necessary to take disciplinary action with a chronic offender, the posted prohibition will support the supervisor's contention that the employee had every reasonable opportunity to know about the rules against personal copying.

Also to be posted are the legal requirements concerning the photocopying of copyrighted material and certain other documents that cannot be legally copied. Despite posted prohibitions against copying copyrighted material, much such material passes through many photocopiers. Nevertheless the posting generally places the legal responsibility for such copying clearly in the hands of the individual who is doing the copying (rather than making the organization responsible). However, in all fairness to individuals who may from time to time put copyrighted material through the machine, it would also be helpful to post the highlights of the "fair use" portion of the United States copyright law that allows limited numbers of copies of certain copyrighted documents to be produced for educational purposes and such.

3) *Control machine access.* The most effective way to control machine access is by the use of key cards or other actuating devices assigned to individual users or departments. These devices turn on the copier—the machine will not run without them—and also count the numbers of copies run so that copying costs may be correctly allocated to the using departments or individuals.

From the point of view of a supervisor of a small- to medium-sized department, it makes sense to have one actuating device for the department in general, ordinarily in the possession of the individual who does most of the department's copying, and perhaps one backup device in the possession of the supervisor.

4) *Use the most economical process.* A shared copy machine or a small machine assigned to a particular department may be more than adequate for short copy runs. However, longer runs of copying are more economical if done on larger, high-volume, high-speed machines ordinarily centralized in print shops or duplicating centers. The matter of which machine to use for which specific copy run can be readily resolved through a simple economic analysis based on actual copying costs. Such analysis might result in a simple posting at a small machine that says something like: "Use this machine to run up to 5 copies. For 6 or more copies, please use the duplicating services department." Guidelines such as the foregoing tend to channel the larger portions of an organization's copying toward more economical copy processes.

5) *Consolidate the bulk of the department's copying with one person.* Consider assigning a single individual to do the majority of the department's copying, perhaps making a "copy run" two or three times each day or as volume or immediate need may dictate. This practice tends to save the time involved when many people make frequent individual trips to the copy machine and also tends to reduce the amount of personal copying that is done.

6) *Run only needed copies.* There is a general tendency to run more copies than are ordinarily needed, primarily because photocopying has become so easy. One should perhaps count the number of copies needed beforehand or at least make a realistic estimate of need, and then consider adding an extra or two in case of need. Because copying is so easy—it takes very little more time and effort to acquire ten copies than it does five—it is far too common to find large numbers of extra copies run "just in case." However, far too many of these extra copies never go anywhere but the trash can (unless—even worse—they go into desks and file cabinets and onto shelves and credenzas, adding to general office clutter and useless storage).

TELEPHONE

The most common causes of excess telephone cost are:

- personal calls;
- inappropriate calls (mail should have been used instead);
- unnecessary telephone equipment.

1) *Personal calls.* Personal telephone calls are wasters of resources on two counts: the direct cost of the calls and the working time of employees that is lost (if such calls are not being made on employees' own time).

Many employees genuinely do not know, and thus need to be advised, that under the majority of most organizations' telephone arrangements even each local call costs a specific amount of money. The days of flat-rate unlimited local calling are rapidly coming to an end, and it is not uncommon for an organization to face a charge of nine or ten cents even for each brief local call that is placed.

It may be periodically necessary to remind employees that there should be no personal use of the telephones. In doing so the supervisor may also have to encourage the organization, through higher management, to assure that public telephones are available for employees to use on their own time.

When it is possible to do so, outside lines should be strictly limited to those specific telephones assigned to those persons or work stations that have a clear need for outside calling. Likewise, direct-dial long distance capability should be strictly limited to those employees who have a clear need to make such calls on a regular basis.

The supervisor should repeatedly assure that all employees know about the organization's prohibition on personal calls, and further must let proven violators know that disciplinary action can result from telephone abuse. As necessary, progressive disciplinary action should be applied fairly and consistently if violations of this basic prohibition continue.

2) *Inappropriate calls.* Consider the case of Mr. Smith, the director of finance in a sizeable hospital. Mr. Smith belonged to three national organizations on behalf of the hospital, and in addition to transacting business relating to these organizations also engaged in other cross-country contacts relatively often. Mr. Smith tended to meet all of his deadline dates; as a rule, exactly on the date he was to have something accomplished or some bit of information transmitted, he reached for the telephone.

If Mr. Smith had adjusted his work habits and allowed time for a letter to travel instead of making a last-minute telephone call he could have saved the organization considerable money. Although he might not have been conscious of doing so, Mr. Smith consumed a fair amount of time on the telephone transacting a single item of business because, when speaking, his thoughts were not nearly as organized or channeled as when he was writing a letter. He was not fully appreciative of the fact that a single $20 long distance telephone call would buy a great deal of letter typing time.

At this point one might be tempted to respond with the latest word on what the average letter costs in secretarial time and all else that goes into it. However, the full "cost" of a letter is not an added out-of-pocket cost for each letter produced. Mr. Smith's secretary, as well as the secretaries of a great many other managers, will generally be there all day every day whether they produce one letter or a half-dozen letters. In this sense the secretary represents a fixed cost. The variable cost of producing each of Mr. Smith's letters generally amounts to no more than the paper and envelope and stamp. However, the $20 charge for Mr. Smith's long distance telephone call is all variable cost—if the call is avoided, $20 is saved.

There are of course times when the telephone is the preferred, if not absolutely necessary, means of communication. However, such is not always the case and we rely too heavily on the telephone to compensate for our lack of an organized, forward-thinking approach to the job. A reasonable amount of planning can eliminate many inappropriate telephone calls. Also, there are other advantages involved in the appropriate use of the mail; a letter provides documentation on one's exact message and reasonable evidence of when the message was transmitted, information that is not available when the telephone is used.

3) *Unnecessary features.* For organizations served by most public or commercial telephone companies, every telephone handset and every additional line on a phone, every button, every light, and every other feature, carries its own monthly charge. These costs recur with every bill even if the features are not used. Therefore, a great deal of care should be taken in assigning lines, buttons, lights, and other features, and even assigning telephone handsets themselves. Once in place many of these items tend to stay in place even if not used; to remove a telephone's feature and remove the feature's monthly charge from the bill generally requires payment of a stiff service charge that often requires years to pay itself back through savings.

The Supervisor and the Telephone Bill

Telephone bills ordinarily associate calls made with the specific calling-line number, so for a department that has its own outside lines calls can be identified with those lines. Each line, that is, each telephone number, can be associated with the number of local calls made, and each specific long distance call made can be identified by the number that was called.

Many supervisors rarely if ever see the telephone bills for their own departments. However, it may be appropriate to ask to see the bill for one's own department. The worst that can happen is that the supervisor, for no reason at all or perhaps for reasons that make little sense, may be denied a chance to see the bill. More likely than not, however, the supervisor can secure the telephone bill for the department. If asked why the bill is requested, one should straightforwardly state that he or she is interested in controllng the department's telephone use and perhaps saving the organization some money.

The supervisor should consider periodically auditing the telephone bill for the department. Questionable charges should be challenged, especially for long distance calls identified with lines not ordinarily used for such calls, or for long distance calls that appear to be excessively long.

Also to be challenged, and indeed investigated until thoroughly satisfactory results are achieved, are calls that appear to have been made by no one in the department. If employees from elsewhere are using the department's telephones the practice should be identified and halted. Also, when great numbers of long distance calls are made and the billing information flows between telephone companies and customers, it is not unusual to find a department charged in error with long distance calls that belong on other bills.

Some employees may misuse the telephone simply without thinking about cost. Certain employees will deliberately misuse telephone service if they are allowed to feel that no one is paying attention to telephone use or that no one cares about telephone use. For example, in one large health care organization no particular attention was paid to telephone costs in most departments—no attention, that is, until the administrator in charge of the emergency department noticed that the department's telephone charges had recently increased by more than $200 per month. Since this represented a dramatic increase over a longstanding, steady level of usage, he sought to satisfy his curiosity about the cause. His investigation revealed that a single evening-shift employee, a person whose date of employment was also about the time when the telephone charges increased, was spending a great deal of available time on the evening shift telephoning family and friends throughout the country. When confronted the employee conceded, after some discussion, that he was aware that telephone calls cost money but that it probably was not much and that the expense had never really crossed his mind.

Although personal long distance calling can always be specifically identified and controlled and should not be allowed to occur, a certain amount of local personal calling is going to take place. As in controlling other elements of nonwage cost, there is no need for the supervisor to go overboard and implement such rigid, authoritarian controls that employee relations problems develop and overall costs are actually increased. However, the supervisor should at least be aware of the level of the telephone bill and any changes it may display, and should periodically audit the bill as he or she might audit any other item of expense. In general, the supervisor should communicate to the staff: telephone service is relatively costly, it exists for conducting the business of the organization, and it should not be used for personal communication.

TRAVEL AND CONFERENCES

The organization that frequently sends people on trips for educational and other purposes should, for the organization as a whole:

• Have a written policy that is available to and fully known by all employees engaging in job-related travel.

- Designate a central travel manager for the organization, or at least provide a central point of approval for the organization's job-related travel.
- If relying on travel agencies, concentrate the organization's business with a single agency that is fully knowledgeable of the organization's policy.
- Be sufficiently organized concerning travel to be able to take advantage of organizational discounts whenever they are available.

Within the individual supervisor's department, the keys to the control of travel and conference costs lie in careful budgeting of such activities and conscientious control of expenditures against the budget. The supervisor should, insofar as possible, budget well in advance according to the needs of the department, considering all known, scheduled trips plus the supervisor's best estimates of other travel and conference needs that are likely to arise.

When granting requests for any particular trip, the supervisor should insist on adherence to any policy limits that may be placed on travel distance. For example, one health care organization requires that conference trips to locations more than 500 miles away receive the approval of the president of the organization. Such policy limits are in place to encourage the supervisor and potential conference attendees to look for closer alternatives to far distant and thus more costly programs.

The supervisor should be supportive of the accounting department and insist on adherence to the organization's policy concerning payment of expenses, insisting on receipts and other required proof of expenditures. Also, the supervisor of a department in a not-for-profit health care organization should assure that each employee who makes an overnight trip within the same state is furnished with a copy of the organization's tax exempt certificate so that sales tax may be avoided on lodging costs.

Finally, although an occasional seminar trip may be considered as a sort of reward for an outstanding employee, conference attendance should never be conferred on an employee simply because it is "your turn to go." Rather, conference attendance should be apportioned in the same manner as any other resource that costs money, primarily as it relates to supporting the needs of the organization.

SUBSCRIPTIONS

The cost of subscriptions may amount to little or nothing for some departments but may be a significant element of cost in certain other departments. As well as including the cost of business-related publications (technical journals and such), this item of nonwage cost also often includes information-service subscriptions, some of which may run into the hundreds of dollars per year. Such information services include multivolume binder sets updated several times per year on the subject of, for example: law as it applies to hospitals or other health care organizations; current law as it applies to labor organizing and active collective bargaining relatonships; tax law and tax regulations; and matters of employment (such as Fair Labor Standard or Equal Employment Opportunity).

Although subscription cost will not be a substantial item for most departments, it nevertheless deserves detailed review at least annually. Once each year, preferably in preparation for beginning the budgeting activity for the coming year, the supervisor or a knowledgeable delegate should:

- Assemble a current list of all active subscriptions coming into the department.
- Solicit staff input on the value of continuing each specific publication, and recommend dropping those that are no longer required or are no longer seen as of value. For example, as a result of a recent such activity a personnel department was able to drop 3 of its 16 annual subscriptions because investigation revealed that these three publications were no longer being used.
- Check with the organization's library to see if any of the publications used in the department are duplicated by library subscriptions, and drop any departmental duplicates that are used seldom enough that a library copy could suffice.
- Attempt to weed out subscription publications which experience has shown duplicate the information provided by other, more appropriate publications.

Every time a subscription bill is received the supervisor should compare it with the active publication list. Various organizations' billing processes being what they are, it is not unusual for bills to keep coming for publications that have been cancelled. A surprising number of business organizations simply pay each incoming invoice out of habit, and this practice often renews publications that certain supervisors have already decided to stop. Also, a fairly common form of mail fraud involves sending large business organizations bills for publications they never receive or that may not even exist. Apparently enough such bills are paid to make this a lucrative form of fraud for a few illegal operators. Therefore, the supervisor should audit all bills and never approve a bill for payment without determining that the publication is received and the department does wish to keep receiving it.

Since publication advertising information may come to any number of employees in the department, it makes sense to have this information channeled through the supervisor or through one designated individual to avoid the possibility of duplicating subscriptions or acquiring subscriptions to inappropriate publications. Many employees have discovered that it is easy simply to return a reply card checking the box instructing someone to "bill organization." However, all such purchases should have routine purchase-requisition approval.

MAILING

Since it is accomplished centrally in most large organizations and even in many small organizations, mailing may not be a concern of the individual department. Many organizations long ago discovered that postage seems to "evaporate" significantly if not centrally monitored. For example, one organization that not long ago went from the practice of using scattered postage meters and loose stamps in a number of different areas to one central mailing function realized a decrease from $101,100 in 1983 to $92,000 in 1984 for postage, despite a five percent increase in mailing volume for 1984 over 1983. Managers of this organization concluded that the difference was due largely to postage lost to personal use and to economies possible through centralization (presorted first class mail and other quantity-mailing advantages).

Since postage is easily diverted for personal use, it is undoubtedly best to centralize mailing for minimum shrinkage and to secure the advantage of quantity mailings that are available to not-for-profit organizations. It may also be advisable to recommend centralizing mailing to maximize the opportunity for other postage-related savings. As an example, consider the study that was suggested by the supervisor of a central transcription department who noted that many items going out to physicians included several in the course of each day going to the same physicians, with many of these physicians located in a medical office building less than two blocks from the hospital.

The study recommended by the transcription supervisor resulted in savings of $23,000 per year, or approximately 25 percent of the hospital's total mailing cost. Since it was possible to mail an average of three items in one envelope for a single stamp, the mail room adopted a practice of consolidating the mail each day for the physicians who were sent most of the mail. In addition, the mail for the nearby physicians' office building was batched and hand delivered once each day. Thus a small amount of attention paid to an item of expense often taken for granted resulted in significant savings.

IT'S ALL MONEY

As suggested at the start of this chapter, the individual department's non-salary budget may not amount to a great deal of money, but variances in this part of the budget can nevertheless make the difference between a positive or negative variance for the entire department. Certainly if a given item is worth spending money for, this item is worth budgeting for. It then follows that if an item is worth budgeting for, the expenditures for this item are worth at least a minimal amount of effort toward control.

NOTE

1. Kenneth A. Johnson and Clifford Neely, "Hospital Economic Forecast," *Hospitals*, October 1, 1983, p. 87.

Chapter 14

Making Equipment Decisions

More people should learn to tell their dollars where to go instead of asking them where they went.

Roger W. Babson

Chapter Objectives

- Delineate the supervisor's responsibility in the selection of capital equipment.
- Reinforce the importance of advance planning for capital purchases through the annual capital budget request.
- Outline the supervisor's role as a primary source of information in major capital expenditure projects.
- Outline a process for the supervisor to follow in making routine capital equipment decisions for the department.

"IS IT IN THE CAPITAL BUDGET?"

The perspective of this chapter is that of the individual supervisor or manager. This perspective must be established at the outset because the role of the individual supervisor in deciding on equipment purchases is often dramatically different from the roles of persons who make the decisions in purchasing, finance, and other administrative functions.

In few cases will the individual supervisor have the sole deciding voice in an equipment purchase. However, almost every supervisor does have, or if lacking such should strive to acquire, some voice in the process.

Regarding relatively large capital equipment expenditures, and in states that have certificate-of-need (CON) legislation in place, the equipment acquisition process necessarily involves administration and the board of directors to a considerable extent. The supervisor remains one primary source of input into a detailed, time-consuming process that is coordinated by administration and is dependent at several steps along the way on outside approvals. Even some expenditures that fall well under the CON threshold (which is different among the states and according to type of application) and that perhaps have not received prior blessing through the organization's budgeting process, frequently require board approval as well as administrative approval. Most organizations observe certain capital expenditure limits dictating that any purchase greater than a certain amount of money must receive, for example, the approval of the finance committee of the board or perhaps the full board of directors.

As well as examining the supervisor's role of providing input in all equipment decisions regardless of size or scope, this chapter will explore the supervisor's active role in recommending equipment purchases that are considerably smaller than the major projects with which capital expenditures are often associated. This approach recognizes that the supervisor will ordinarily see most of the action regarding capital equipment acquisition, such as typewriters, copiers, microcomputers, other office equipment and furniture, and perhaps relatively small pieces of clinical equipment.

As far as possible, it is advisable to plan the department's capital purchases well in advance through the department's annual budget. The amount of capital funds available within a given year is limited organization-wide, and such funds are usually apportioned according to the need. One of the most common responses a supervisor can receive to a request for a piece of equipment is, "Is it in the capital budget?" Since demands for equipment throughout the organization usually far exceed the reach of the dollars available, the supervisor ordinarily has to get in line with not only a request but also a solid justification for the purchase.

There is almost always a considerable amount of competition for available capital budget dollars. Indeed it is not unusual for the sum of all capital budget requests throughout the organization, admittedly often much of a wish list, to amount to more than double the available capital dollars. Since capital funds are finite in amount and limited in supply, the organization's overall capital needs must be planned.

Ideally, capital expenditure planning begins before the preparation of the next year's budget. If the institution's annual budgeting exercise begins in September, for example, it is wise to begin no later than June or July to prepare to justify the purchase of equipment desired for the coming year.

Two alternate but partially overlapping paths will be pursued in the balance of this chapter, considering:

1. major capital equipment requiring approval (but not necessarily CON), the requests for which originate with the supervisor;
2. other (and generally lesser) capital equipment, requests originating with the supervisor and requiring the organization's normal administrative approval.

MAJOR CAPITAL EQUIPMENT

Large equipment purchases are of less concern to the individual supervisor than those that originate solely with the supervisor. Although large purchases are important to the organization as a whole, the individual supervisor is but one of many people who bear some measure of responsibility for such projects. Even though a project requiring major equipment purchases may occasionally originate with the supervisor, there are always numerous other persons who become involved and there are group processes and outside processes over which the supervisor has little or no control.

One key area of supervisory involvement in major equipment purchases is gathering and assembling the information required for the complete analysis of proposals and the potential allocation of capital funds. Depending on the scope of any undertaking and thus on the depth and extent of the supervisor's involvement, the supervisor may be called on to provide pieces of the following information:

1) *Reason for request.* A major equipment purchase is usually requested for one or a combination of the following reasons:

- The purchase is required by regulation or accreditation. Equipment must often be purchased to bring the institution into compliance with regulations and thus permit continued legal operation, or such a purchase is often encouraged by the spectre of loss of accreditation. In most such cases the requirement of regulation or accreditation is sufficient justification for the purchase.

- The equipment may be requested to replace existing equipment. Obviously in such cases the justification for the request will proceed along the lines of demonstrating why and how the existing equipment is no longer adequate.
- The request calls for the addition of new equipment to perform a function not previously performed. Since this ordinarily involves the provision of a new service, the justification of the equipment purchase is but a part (although a significant part) of the economic and clinical justification for adding the new service.

2) *Department priority.* If the department is involved in a number of capital equipment requests, each should have a specific place on a priority listing of requests. In turn, the organization as a whole will usually develop a rank-order listing of organization-wide priorities.

3) *General assessment of need.* Assessment of need is ordinarily the narrative portion of a capital budget request and should state what is being requested, not only of the specific piece of equipment but, as appropriate, the entire project or undertaking of which the equipment is to be part. Overall this narrative should identify the function or concern within the organization that the request is intended to address, state whether this is a proposed change in treatment modality, the adoption of new or improved technology, the reduction of medical complications, or the improvement of quality in general, and indicate the savings of time, the reduction of costs, or the potential increase in revenue to be gained.

The narrative should explain why the requesters believe that the equipment being asked for is the most efficient and effective way of performing the function or addressing the concern that triggered the request. Also, it is helpful if the narrative attempts to deal with the potential usefulness or applicability of the proposed purchase under present circumstances, within the short run (up to one year in the future), and within the longer run, looking perhaps four or five years into the future.

4) *Assessment of clinical implications.* It is often advisable to proceed beyond the general assessment of need to an additional, clinically oriented assessment of the likely impact of the new equipment or service on both patients and staff. This amounts to an educated attempt to say whether various clinical outcomes would be different than at present if the proposed project is approved and implemented and monitored over a period of time. This assessment of clinical implications ordinarily involves projection of the likely impact, if any, of the proposed budget on length of stay, procedure time, rates of readmission, occurrence of complications, levels of ancillary utilization,

levels of occupancy, utilization of outpatient versus inpatient services, and the comfort and safety of patients or staff or both.

In this section of the evaluation it is also important to bring to light any known or likely emerging technological changes that stand to alter the direction of the project in the foreseeable future. For example, if one were now starting on a two-year approval process for buying a piece of major equipment knowing that emerging technology could make this desired equipment obsolete within two to three years, other alternatives for performing the function or providing the service might be pursued.

5) *Personnel requirements.* For any request for major capital equipment it is necessary, as part of the assessment of the overall project, to identify the skills of the people who will be expected to operate the equipment and to enumerate the costs associated with such personnel. Any new personnel should be identified at least by skill level and pay grade and work status (full-time, or part-time for some specific number of hours per week). This assessment should consider, in addition to the possibility of added personnel in the department, the use of existing personnel at present grade levels or the need to upgrade existing personnel. All cost information related to personnel should be reflected in the following section.

6) *Tentative cost information.* At this stage of the process all cost information is tentative. Detailed specifications have not yet been developed and formal applications have not been created. To be applied only as guidelines, but nevertheless to be as accurate as possible given the early stages of the project, are quotations or estimates concerning:

- Total acquisition cost of the equipment. This includes not only the purchase price of the equipment but also the costs of transporting the equipment to the point of use and installing and preparing to operate the equipment. In accounting practice, transportation cost, usually a separately enumerated item, is considered part of the cost of acquisition and thus must be capitalized as such. Equipment installation costs are also capital costs; these are often significant when one considers the construction work and related effort that must take place to bring a new piece of equipment to its point of use and to prepare it to operate.
- Estimated useful life of the equipment must be provided. Whether subsequent financial analysis demonstrates the proposed project to be attractive or unattractive frequently revolves around the number of years the equipment is expected to perform its intended function.
- The estimated annual personnel costs must be provided from the information provided in step 5. For an analysis that will be as accurate as

possible, this should represent added personnel costs only, the incremental costs to be borne only when and if this equipment is put into service. (In other words, if the new equipment is to be operated by existing personnel at their existing rates of pay, there are no incremental personnel costs.)

- Estimated costs of materials and supplies necessitated by the equipment, and, as a separate figure, the estimated annual cost of service and maintenance for the equipment. Both of these figures are required for preliminary analysis of the economic feasibility of the project.
- The estimated annual volume of work to be served by the equipment. This is critical information that will ultimately play an important role in determining whether the project is or is not economically feasible.

In addition to the foregoing six categories of information, it will be helpful to provide any additional justification for the project that may be available. For instance, should the request involve the replacement of existing equipment, it would make sense to provide as much information as possible as to why the present equipment is no longer adequate.

Should it be the supervisor who is initiating the request and supplying the information as far as a major capital expenditure is concerned, the supervisor is actually, at this stage, "requesting a request." That is, since numerous other managers and their functions have to become involved in assessing the feasibility of the proposed undertaking and providing input to the formal request for capital expenditure, the supervisor is, at best, providing only the trigger for the request process. Nevertheless this is often the supervisor's most vital role relative to a proposed major capital expenditure. Once a proposal has evolved to the status of a formal request, the supervisor is then one of a sizeable team, all the members of which have various responsibilities.

OTHER CAPITAL EQUIPMENT

Most of the equipment with which the individual supervisor will become involved is of lesser dollar value than implied by the discussion in the preceding section. Also, most of the equipment of interest to many supervisors is nonclinical. Foremost among items for the supervisor's consideration are office and business equipment, kitchen equipment, tools, and such. Most of these items are intended for use by the departments of the requesting supervisors in fulfillment of these departments' basic functions.

Very often such equipment requests are essentially approved when the department's capital budget for the coming year is approved. Therefore it makes sense for the supervisor to do the best possible job of justifying the need for desired equipment at the time the capital budget is prepared. In preparing the justification for acquiring a piece of equipment, the supervisor would normally include the same kinds of information as delineated in the previous section—the reason for the request, the department's priority, the general assessment of need, the assessment of clinical implications, if any, the personnel requirements, and cost information as completely as possible.

Using Internal Resources

Virtually every established health care organization has a policy requiring all requests for quotations and related information to go through the purchasing department. In addition, in many organizations the first purchasing criterion is that items requested must be approved budget items.

For detailed information on equipment manufacturers, model capacities, and prices, the individual supervisor should ask the purchasing department. One may have pre-existing ideas about manufacturer, make, model, and such, but the purchasing department may have other more preferable alternatives to offer. The purchasing department is ordinarily considerably faster than the individual supervisor at locating up-to-date information on any kind of equipment, so there is little point for the supervisor to attempt to duplicate a function performed more efficiently by others. Also, there is little point for the supervisor to go about collecting and retaining catalogues and price lists. Purchasing has information on alternatives and is more likely to have current price information (price lists, especially, change so often that any list the supervisor may retain is sure to be out of date in some respects within a few months).

For certain kinds of purchases, the purchasing department may recommend one "standard" or may at least recommend a narrow range of choices based on experience and other considerations. The organization may be able to obtain price breaks based on quantity, or may be recommending specific choices based on various suppliers' records of reliability or promptness of service. Purchasing may also recommend a fairly narrow range of proven choices because of the economy and ease of administration of service contracts. For example, an organization may use only two or three different makes of typewriter, as opposed to allowing two dozen different brand names into the organization, because two or three master service contracts are far more economical and easily administered than two dozen different ones.

Again depending on the size of the organization and the organization's policies regarding purchasing, a purchase request for equipment may also require a supervisor to:

- Secure a detailed cost estimate from engineering services concerning the installation of the equipment, including all construction modfications and electrical and plumbing and other utility work that must be accomplished. Ordinarily the estimate must be approved by administration before submission.

- Secure biomedical engineering review and approval for equipment that may eventually be serviced by the institution's biomedical engineering function.
- Present evidence to the effect that specifications of the proposed equipment have been reviewed and approved for employee and patient safety considerations by the safety manager, and that the equipment appears to conform to all existing safety regulations.

Deciding What to Ask For

The supervisor should consider several important steps to the extent necessary to decide on what particular piece of equipment to buy.

1) *Delineate task specifications.* One must specify the kind of function to be performed by the equipment and provide, as accurately as possible, all of the quality requirements of the function and all requirements for quantity of task output. The supervisor should ordinarily know what the needs are regarding quality. Regarding quantity, however, it is often necessary to rely on reasonable estimates. Because quantity of output should take into consideration projected future needs over the estimated life of the equipment as well as present estimated life of the equipment and present needs, some estimating is inevitable.

2) *Identify several products that will do the job.* Through the purchasing department, through other managers, and through other available sources, the supervisor should identify a number of products that will do the job identified in the first step. This involves determining pieces of equiment that will produce the quality level required in the performance of the task and that can provide the quantity of output necessary to meet present and anticipated needs. It is impossible to say specifically how many different products the supervisor should identify during this step. If the equipment in question is special-purpose equipment, manufactured by only two or three suppliers, perhaps two or three alternatives are all that can be located. However, for fairly common departmental capital equipment such as typewriters, photocopiers, microcomputers, and such, there are a considerable number of suppliers available so the supervisor might identify five or six appropriate alternatives.

3) *Apply constraints.* It is often necessary for the supervisor to acknowledge constraints that establish limitations on some of the alternatives identified for consideration. Such constraints are often economic in nature, existing

in the form of dollar limits on certain kinds of expenditures as established during the budgeting process or arising from economic necessity. For example, if it is an organization's policy to govern capital expenditures by approving projected expenditures in the capital budgeting process, then the supervisor who has budget approval to spend $4,000 on a microcomputer cannot spend more than that even though he might have concluded, since budget time, that a particular $5,000 computer is the one that is really needed. Thus in many organizations it is important that the supervisor's capital budget submissions be as detailed and as well thought out as possible so that all realistic options remain open. However, a capital budget item approved in the fall of the coming year is not necessarily guaranteed. A budget is generated in advance of the time period to which it applies, and the applicable time period, when it arrives, can bring a turn of events that adversely affects the organization's overall finances and can dictate that certain capital expenditures will amount to less than budgeted or will perhaps not occur at all.

Occasionally one will also encounter constraints of a political nature. Perhaps because of previous unsatisfactory experiences or a generally poor record of relations with a supplier, the organization may have adopted a policy (often unwritten) of dealing with that firm infrequently if at all. Perhaps there are personality differences between the supplier's representatives and the institution's decision makers that make the decision makers less favorably inclined toward that supplier.

There may also be physical constraints that have to be taken into account. Rarely are such constraints absolute, but they are often sufficiently important as to boost the cost of some alternatives to unreasonble levels. As previously noted, the legitimate cost of acquiring a piece of equipment also includes the cost of installation. This includes the cost of any modifications or alterations necessary to accommodate the equipment, and these added costs can readily render an otherwise attractive alternative unreasonable. For example, one relatively small organization identified a fairly unique constraint on their selection of a new copy machine and worked this into their specifications: The new machine could not be more than 29 inches wide. The machine was to replace an older machine that had essentially been built into a small, fully occupied utility room much as an automatic dishwasher would be built into a kitchen. It would have been physically possible to accommodate a wider machine but doing so would have required either breaking through a load-bearing, plumbing-filled wall on one side or relocating an electrical input line and breaker box on the other side, effectively more than doubling the acquisition cost of any machine more than 29 inches wide.

In general, the consideration of constraints as an intermediate stage of the evaluation process is intended to weed out those otherwise workable choices that are rendered impossible because of absolute constraints or that are rendered impractical because of known limiting or restricting factors.

4) *Compare the realistic alternatives.* This is a two-fold process in which the supervisor should:

- Attempt to zero in on the best of the known choices.
- Develop a thorough justification for the choice (or refine and update the existing justification if such had been provided during the capital budgeting process).

The selection of the apparent best choice and the development of the justification should take the form of a comparative analysis of all reasonable alternatives through both objective economic analysis and subjective assessment of intangible factors.

The economic analysis should take into account all costs of acquiring and using the equipment, including:

- acquisition, which, as noted, includes purchase price, cost of shipping, and total cost of installation;
- estimated cost of all materials and supplies to be consumed in the operation of the equipment;
- costs of additional personnel required or cost of essential upgrading of existing personnel;
- cost, if any, of training personnel to operate the equipment;
- estimated cost of maintenance, service, and repairs;
- other applicable costs such as insurance premiums, license costs, various fees, additional power and other utility requirements.

Since different pieces of equipment often have different anticipated life spans, it is difficult to evaluate several alternatives unless they are placed on a common footing for analysis. Thus it is best to develop the economic comparison of alternatives on the basis of equivalent annual costs, that is, the cost of owning and operating each alternative on a per-year basis. (The following section presents a simple example of economic analysis on the basis of equivalent annual cost.)

However, economic analysis alone is often not enough to sway a supervisor's decision, especially when, as may be the case, two or more choices prove nearly equal in dollar value. One must proceed to consider the intangible factors associated with each alternative and thus inject an element of judgment into the decision-making process. The intangibles to be considered in most of the supervisor's equipment decisions may include:

- the reputation of the potential supplier, perhaps including the relative weight of the brand name of the equipment;

- the perception of the supervisor and others of the relative reliability of a particular supplier's equipment;
- the readiness of access to the supplier's service function, and the supervisor's and others' perception of the firm's reliability and responsiveness concerning service;
- the relative stability of the organization's relationship with the firm's sales representatives.

In general, the intangible factors in such a decision all add up in contributing to a "gut feeling" that inclines toward yes, no, or indifference. There is nothing scientific about the assessment of the intangible factors, but they nevertheless need to be considered. A decision made solely on the basis of economics is not a thoroughly considered decision. Numbers do not decide; it is people who decide. For a decision to stand a chance of being a good decision, the supervisor must be able to feel reasonably confident that it is a good decision under the circumstances.

5) *Recommend a choice.* It is often helpful to submit not only one's best decision as a first choice but also to offer a second best along with a reason for this order of preferred alternatives. It may be helpful to provide the dollars-and-cents results of one's complete comparative economic analysis along with a narrative description of the recommendation including the judgmental assessment of intangible factors.

Example: The Copy Machine

Consider the tasks of a supervisor who is preparing to decide on a new copy machine to replace the department's worn-out machine. This supervisor has taken into account all known and estimated photocopy requirements for the coming several years and has identified at least six copy machines that would appropriately serve the department's purposes. However, the constraints on the decision situation (the outer limits of that which is possible or practical) have ruled out three otherwise appropriate choices, so the supervisor is left with three machines for direct comparison. Further, according to the way their manufacturers do business, two of the three machines must be purchased outright but the third machine can be either purchased or leased. Therefore, this supervisor has four alternatives to consider.

Exhibit 14-1, Pertinent Information on Copy Machines A, B, C, is a summary of the economic information required by the supervisor in performing an economic comparison. Since the alternative machines have different estimated useful lives, it is not possible to compare alternatives in terms of total cost or any particular one-time cost. A reasonable basis for comparison, as already suggested, is the cost of possessing and using each machine on a per year basis.

Exhibit 14-1 Pertinent Information on Copy Machines A, B, and C

```
Machine A — Acquisition cost ........................................ $ 2,800
            Estimated useful life ................................... 4 years
            Paper and supplies ..................................... $ 2,400/yr
            Operator training (one-time cost) ....................... $   400
            Service contract....................................... $   500/yr

Machine B — Acquisition cost ........................................ $ 3,750
            Estimated useful life ................................... 5 years
            Paper and supplies ..................................... $ 2,200/yr
            Operator training (one-time cost) ....................... $   400
            Service contract....................................... $   500/yr

Machine C — Acquisition cost (purchase)............................. $ 3,000
            Acquisition cost (lease) ............................... $ 1,400/yr
            Estimated useful life ................................... 3 years
            Paper and supplies ..................................... $ 1,800/yr
            Operator training ...................................... (none)
            Service contract if purchase ........................... $   400/yr
            Service contract if lease............................... (no cost)
```

This example should suggest that even so-called factual data are often not nearly as factual as they may seem. The dollar figures of Exhibit 14-1 are to be trusted, but information is presented other than specific dollar amounts. The estimated useful life is just that, estimated. Surely it is based on some historical information that relates life to usage, and just as surely it has some connection with the time period over which such equipment may be depreciated for accounting purposes. However, one has no guarantee that, for example, machine A will last precisely four years as estimated; it may last six or seven years in normal service, or it may break down between the second and third year, and if either of these occurrences was known for certain the economic comparison of alternatives might change considerably. Thus one must simply go with available guidelines and use the best information available. Also appearing as an estimate in the information is the cost of paper and supplies. Paper and supply usage are based on volume, and future volume is necessarily an estimate. However, one is on firmer ground with this figure than with the estimated useful life because the same estimated volume is included in the cost of paper and supplies for all three alternatives so if reality proves it to be wrong, it is consistently wrong for all alternatives and thus has a lesser impact on the overall analysis.

Exhibit 14-2 displays a simple comparison of the equivalent annual costs of the three machines. Four alternatives are available: A, B, and C as an outright purchase, and C under a lease agreement. Thus on the basis of economics alone, the third alternative, acquiring machine C through purchase, emerges as the most economical. However, such economic analysis does not dictate the choice but simply gives a certain amount of weight to the purchase of machine C in overall consideration of the problem. It could perhaps turn out that if the manufacturer of machine C had a poor reputation for service, or that if numerous other users were dissatisfied with the machines made by the manufacturer of machine C, the supervisor might legitimately consider that the potential problems acquired by buying machine C might not be worth the nominal savings in dollars. However, if the assessment of intangibles is satisfactory for the purchase of machine C and is essentially the same for all alternatives, the purchase of machine C is a good common sense choice.

One would pay more attention to the economic analysis if the gap between the winner and the others were significant. However, even when all alternatives come out relatively close to each other in equivalent annual cost— and in the example the $500 per year gap between the costliest and the least expensive is not great—one has at least discovered that the alternatives are essentially a toss up economically and can then proceed to give more weight to the consideration of tangible factors.

A significant element of judgment remains in such a decision despite all economic analysis. There is no such commodity as perfect information in any decision situation; if there were, the result would be a foregone conclusion and there would be no decision to make. Thus there is always an element of uncertainty, a legitimate doubt as to whether a decision made is the correct one. Likewise, in such decisions there is always an element of risk, that is, there is always something to be lost if the decision is the incorrect one. As long as uncertainty and risk exist, it is necessary to apply some degree of human judgment.

Exhibit 14-2 Equivalent Annual Cost Comparison: Copy Machines A, B, & C

	A	B	C (Buy)	C (Lease)
Annualized acquisition cost (includes shipping and installation)	$ 700	$ 750	$ 1,000	$ 1,400
Paper and supplies	2,400	2,200	1,800	1,800
Operator training	100	80	—	—
Excess copy cost over agreement	—	—		400
Service contract	500	500	400	—
Equivalent cost per year	$ 3,700	$ 3,530	$ 3,200	$ 3,600

In making equipment selection decisions, as in making most managerial decisions, the task is one of limiting uncertainty as much as possible and thus reducing risk, and deciding through the application of judgment. Consider the same supervisor making the same decision simply by shooting from the hip. If the purchasing manager were to line up three machines and ask the supervisor which was preferred and the supervisor were to simply point and say, "I'll take the blue one," the simple probability that the choice represents the correct decision is 33 percent (in other words, the odds are one in three of making the best choice on a random basis). However, through economic comparison of the alternatives plus thoughtful assessment of all intangible factors, it might be possible to improve one's probability of making the "correct" decision to perhaps 75 or 80 percent. Thus in approaching such decisions systematically the supervisor is simply improving the odds to which he or she is exposed.

SOPHISTICATED ECONOMIC ANALYSIS

The approach to economic analysis presented in the copy machine example, the use of equivalent annual cost, is the simplest way of looking at the economics of alternative choices, but in many instances it is fully adequate to the supervisor's needs. Occasionally, however, and especially in borderline cases and on projects of considerable dollar value, much more detailed analysis is required. In-depth financial analysis often considers the time value of money and a number of additional factors. When capital budget dollars are tight and there is a great deal of competition for this money among more projects than could possibly be funded, the organization will take steps to make sure that the best choices are made as to where the dollars are placed. Also, when times are tight financially, those projects that show the most promise of enhancing revenue have an automatic edge over projects that simply support the present income stream.

In further analysis it may also be necessary to consider the payback period of each project. The payback period is that length of time, usually expressed in years or fractional parts of years, required for an investment to pay for itself through increased output, increased revenue, or cost savings. All other factors being equal, the shorter the payback period the more attractive the investment.

If capital dollars are borrowed, there are the not inconsiderable costs of interest to reckon with in the analysis. This is the time value of money. If money must be borrowed to pay for a particular piece of equipment or if the equipment must be bought on a time payment basis, the actual cost of interest must enter into the economic comparison. Even if the organization is in a position to pay cash for a piece of equipment, opportunity cost must still be reckoned with. Since money that is not used for one purpose can be used for another, the earnings foregone on alternative use of the funds—the opportunity cost—is often considered in the economic analysis. For example, if the $3,200 that might be paid for machine C were not spent for that machine but were instead invested at 12 percent, the 12 percent compound interest on that money for the life of machine C would be the opportunity cost of that alternative.

Occasionally cash flow problems can affect the choice of which piece of equipment to purchase. Again referring to the example, the purchase of machine C may emerge as the best alternative economically. But if this machine purchase was not budgeted—assume this is a replacement machine needed because the old machine, which was supposed to have lasted longer, simply died and had to be replaced—there might not be money available. If no funds remained available to meet an unplanned need, then the best way to solve the copy machine decision might be to lease machine C to provide the minimum impact on cash flow. The purchase of machine C might be the most logical choice, and it might appear to be a bargain. However, to paraphrase an anonymous saying, "A bargain's not a bargain if you can't pay the price."

If ever it appears necessary to go beyond simple equivalent annual cost analysis, the supervisor should ask for assistance from the organization's finance section. Finance is far better equipped through knowledge and experience to deal with such matters, and they usually have computer software available that will quickly run time-value comparisons when fed the appropriate data. The average nonfinancial supervisor would not ordinarily be expected to handle the sophisticated economic analysis that may be necessary only occasionally. Indeed it is not the responsibility of the supervisor always to know all of the answers; rather, it is the supervisor's responsiblity to know where to go for the appropriate answers when needed.

A WORD ABOUT OBSOLESCENCE

In these days of technological advancement in all aspects of business, in the delivery of health care services and otherwise, the piece of equipment purchased today is likely to be superseded next month or next year by a new generation of equipment that will perform the same function better, faster, or more cheaply. Often those who supply work organizations with equipment would have us believe that acquisition of the "new and improved" model is essential to our continued efficient operation. We are frequently told that what we are using is now obsolete. However, there is more than one kind of obsolescence.

Much equipment in the modern health care organization is indeed technically obsolete, meaning that there is now something available that is technologically better and will in some way perform the function better. However, for a piece of equipment to be truly obsolete it must be functionally obsolete, that is, it will no longer do the job it is intended to do.

Functional obsolescence is true obsolescence. When a piece of equipment can no longer perform its function, it is either because the equipment has deteriorated or the function has changed. Consider again the copy machine example. Assume that the organization purchased machine C, and that 15 months later the sales representative returns with the news that machine C is obsolete and machine NIC (New and Improved C) is available. Machine NIC will generate copies 25 percent faster than machine C, so machine C is indeed obsolete (technically obsolete). However, examination of machine C in use reveals that copy volumes have been occurring much as expected and that only an average 50 percent of machine C's capacity is utilized. Copy quality has remained the same and quality requirements are unchanged. Thus machine C is not functionally obsolete because it will still perform the function it was intended to perform at essentially the same cost.

In short, that which is branded as obsolete is not necessarily functionally obsolete. Generally, as long as a piece of equipment is doing the job it is intended to do, there is no point in changing simply to have all of the "latest features." It is only when all of the latest features add up to bankable cost savings that the purchase of new equipment is justified, or when the old equipment is truly functionally obsolete, that it makes sense to change.

Chapter 15

Energy Management at the Supervisor's Level

Roughly speaking, half of all the energy consumed by man in the past 2,000 years has been consumed in the last one hundred.

Alvin Toffler

Chapter Objectives

- Establish the extent to which the individual supervisor can influence expenditures for energy (which can fall in the range of three to five percent of an institution's budget).
- Provide guidelines applicable to every supervisor in promoting and achieving energy conservation.
- Furnish detailed conservation checklists for high-energy-using departments (food service and laundry).
- Delineate the supervisor's key role in establishing an energy-conscious attitude in the employee group.

Energy management may be defined as the continuous active consideration of efficient and effective energy usage in the operation of facilities.[1] Energy management may also be described as the integration of energy cost and conservation factors with the process of planning for new construction or planning the modification of existing facilities.

Although it should be apparent that there is much that can be done in the average health care institution regarding energy management, it should be equally apparent that the power of the individual supervisor to influence appreciably the overall organization's use of energy is limited. Energy management is most productively pursued within an organization-wide energy management program of which each individual supervisor is but one of many active participants. If the organization does have a formal energy management program, the advice contained in this chapter is superfluous. However, if there is no overall energy management program, this chapter's advice becomes useful in helping the supervisor control a portion of the institution's energy expenditures. Although the absence of an organization-wide energy management program severely limits the number of energy-saving steps the supervisor can take, there nevertheless remain a sufficient number of potential energy-saving options open to the supervisor to justify attention to energy conservation.

Before the early 1970s there was little recognized need for an organized approach to energy management. A few common sense controls were applied to energy as they were also applied to other resources costing money, but energy was of relatively minor importance in the complex process of managing a health care institution. Energy was essentially regarded as coming from a bottomless well; no matter how much was used, the well was always full and flowing and the cost was always reasonable if not inconsequential.

During 1970 the majority of the health care institutions in the country were spending considerably less than one percent of their annual budgets on energy. However, ten years later, in 1980, the share of the average institution's budget devoted to energy had risen to the range of three to five percent.[2] It was of course the oil embargo of 1973–1974 that first raised the nation's consciousness regarding the existence of very real limitations on energy supplies, a consciousness that was renewed and intensified by the next oil crisis that occurred near the end of the 1970s.

By 1979, "We need energy management" had become a rallying cry of organization management nationwide. Still feeling the shock of having their annual energy costs multiply three, four, or five times over, management groups in all kinds of organizations were heaping much tribute on the necessity of energy management. But much of this tribute proved to be verbal only; many organizations that established committees and adopted formal energy management programs have since either abandoned their programs entirely

or allowed them to grind to a halt on their own. Once the jolt of dramatically increased energy costs was absorbed and these higher costs began to gain
long-run acceptance born of reality, and organization's patterns of budgeting
and spending adapted to this new reality, the perceived need for energy
management lost much of its urgency. In the face of modest but steady
declines in energy costs through 1984 and 1985, energy management as a formal undertaking lost even more of its appeal. Having reached a point at which
the "outrageous" energy prices of a few years earlier had finally been accepted as "normal," price reductions began to be viewed as genuine decreases
from an accepted level.

The fact remains, however, that the average institution will now spend three
percent or more of its budget on energy compared with less than one percent
in 1970. Although the crises have apparently been weathered and the shock
waves of sudden change have been absorbed, it is still true, for example,
that a gallon of heating oil today costs about three times as much as in early
1973. Regardless of what happens to energy supplies and prices in the coming few years, it remains unlikely that energy costs will ever return to anywhere
near their pre-1973 levels. In other words, we can accept the likelihood that
the days of cheap energy are gone for good. Never again will we be able to
regard energy as endless in supply and relatively inconsequential in cost.

The ultimate goal of energy management in the health care institution
should be to consume the least possible amount of energy to perform the
institution's functions adequately. Even in the absence of an organization-
wide program, it can still be the individual supervisor's goal to consume the
least possible amount of energy in performing the department's functions.
However, this goal must be pursued in realistic recognition of those energy
expenditures the supervisor can indeed control or influence and those energy
uses over which the supervisor has no control.

ENERGY CONSERVATION OPPORTUNITIES[3]

The points presented in the listings that follow combine information and
advice concerning: what to look for in the way of energy conservation opportunities; what one's investigations may reveal; and what specific actions
might be considered to generate energy savings. Most of the emphasis is on
no-cost and low-cost opportunities that the supervisor can implement within
the department and low-cost opportunities that may be implemented by the
organization's maintenance department upon the supervisor's request. The
supervisor does not directly control the institution's major energy-consuming
systems. Neither is it ordinarily possible to identify actual energy consumption and cost within a particular department. Consider, for example, the cost
of electricity: The institution as a whole will have perhaps only one or at

the most a very few electric meters, and it is not possible to identify a specific department's electrical usage without installing relatively expensive, individual check meters.

The energy management opportunities available to the supervisor are generally of three types:

1. Those suggesting the development of procedures or end-use instructions. This primarily involves the development and dissemination of guidance in the use of systems or devices so they may be used in an energy-efficient manner.
2. Those calling for inspection and correction on an as-needed basis. This suggests that as certain conditions are encountered, routine adjustments or corrections should be made.
3. Those calling for the modification of existing devices or installation of energy improvements. These opportunities deal with modification or upgrading of certain kinds of equipment, or addition of devices or materials to enhance energy conservation.

To work with the employee group in attempting to conserve energy the supervisor can consider the following concerns.

General Heating and Cooling System Operating Practices

To the extent that the supervisor is able to do so (that is, depending on the availability of individual thermostats and other separate controls for the department), the supervisor can develop procedures or end-use instructions calling for employees to:

- Adjust thermostats of sill-height electric heaters so that heat generated is just sufficient to prevent cool downdrafts from reaching the floor.
- Close window drapes and shades on days during the heating season when the sun is not shining. This will reduce heat loss by radiation to the cool window surface.
- Close outside air dampers during the first and last hours of occupancy and during peakload operating periods (in noncritical areas only).
- Close supply registers and radiators and reduce thermostat settings when appropriate.
- Cool noncritical areas to no lower than 78 °F when occupied. Begin precooling operations so that area temperature is 80 °F by the time occupants arrive.
- Discontinue the heating and cooling of storage areas containing materials not affected by temperature variations.

- Discontinue the heating and cooling of garages and dock and platform areas.
- Heat offices and other noncritical areas to 68 °F when they are occupied and 60 °F when unoccupied. Begin preheating so that such areas reach 65 °F by the time the first occupants arrive, and turn off the heat during the final hour of occupancy.
- Operate self-contained units (such as window or through-the-wall air conditioners) only when needed.
- Operate room cooling fans at reduced speeds during mild weather to reduce the cooling effect of moving air.
- Reduce the use of heating and cooling systems in areas that are infrequently used or used only for brief periods.
- Reduce internal heat generation as much as possible during the cooling season by keeping the use of lights, equipment, and other heat sources to the essential minimum.
- Turn off portable space heaters and fans when not needed.
- Turn off humidification equipment when an entire structure is temporarily closed (for instance, an office building unused on weekends).
- Turn off all exhaust fans in noncritical areas when they are not required.
- Utilize an equipment operating checklist for personnel using various areas before and after regular hours so that no energy-using systems will inadvertently be left running when not needed.

Regarding heating and cooling units and controls and related equipment, the supervisor and the department's employees can also:

- Periodically ensure that routine preventive maintenance and cleaning of equipment are being performed. Should any equipment appear to have been missed or inadvertently excluded from preventive maintenance processes, the supervisor can request that appropriate action be taken.
- Assure that heating and cooling units are free from obstructions that would hamper their operation and assure that all heat transfer surfaces are kept clean for most efficient operation.
- Periodically check for air leaks around window-mounted or through-the-wall units and request appropriate caulking and weatherstripping as needed.
- Immediately report to the maintenance department any equipment that appears to be functioning improperly and any heating and cooling controls that do not appear to be operating as intended.
- Consider the use of locking covers on thermostats to prevent occupants from adjusting settings in areas where altered settings may, for example, unbalance an entire building's system.

Ventilation and Exhaust

Develop procedures or end-use instructions to:

- Specify when exhaust hoods in laboratories, laundries, kitchens, and the like should be used or not used.
- Instruct personnel to close outdoor air dampers during the first and last hours of occupancy in noncritical areas.

Further, the supervisor should request of maintenance that all outdoor air dampers be periodically inspected for proper operation and that filters be cleaned or replaced as necessary.

Transmission

Since heat is transmitted through the majority of solid substances, one should remain aware of potential heat loss through transmission. The primary medium of heat transfer in the typical structure is glass, so the windows deserve most of the supervisor's attention. During the cooling season it makes sense to utilize indoor shading devices efffectively, such as drapes or blinds that are capable of reducing the heat gain from direct sunlight as much as 50 percent. During the heating season, it is advisable to close all indoor shading devices at night to reduce heat loss through windows. Further, it is suggested that all unused and unneeded windows be thermally sealed with opaque or translucent insulating material.

Infiltration

Infiltration refers to the passage of heat through the cracks. Thus most air infiltration occurs in and around doors, windows, and other openings in exterior surfaces such as those created for exhaust fans or through-the-wall air conditioning units. One should periodically inspect for cracked or broken windowpanes, worn, broken, or missing weatherstripping, and misaligned window latches, and request that such deficiencies be corrected. Additional suggestions for controlling infiltration may include:

- posting a label at each operable window instructing occupants to avoid opening windows while the building is being heated or cooled;
- posting a reminder on each door leading outdoors or into unconditioned space advising users to close the door;

• requesting maintenance to look into the possibility of rehanging misaligned doors, repairing door closers that are found to be operating improperly, and replacing worn door seals and weatherstripping where necessary.

Lighting

A great deal of the control of lighting rests with dissemination of information to the work group and creation of a group attitude toward energy conservation. Thus it may be necessary to embark on a campaign of encouraging the use of certain lights only when needed and maintain this campaign until the habit of turning off unused lights has become ingrained. Also, the supervisor should assure that all reflecting surfaces are clean so as to assure maximum lighting efficiency.

The supervisor will do well to request an engineering survey of illumination levels in the department. Before the people who run organizations and the people who design physical facilities became energy conscious, many facilities were overilluminated. It is not unusual to find certain areas (mostly in facilities built before the mid-1970s) that are provided with double the amount of lighting required for normal human business activity. Some organizations have solved this problem in certain areas by taking every second ceiling fixture out of service. Also, since much of the current trend in workplace lighting is toward individual lights at desks and other work stations, it is often possible to save considerable electrical power by drastically cutting back on general area lighting and supplementing with individual workplace lighting.

Regarding the use of electrical power in general, it may be helpful to disseminate end-use instructions through letters, memos, personal contacts, and other means urging personnel to turn off all electrical equipment when not in use. Such equipment would include space heaters (which draw a considerable amount of current), portable fans, typewriters, calculators and computer terminals, coffee pots, and so on.

Hot and Cold Water

Should the supervisor's physical area of responsibility include some elements of the facility's water supply system, it would make sense to inspect those system elements periodically and call for the repair of all apparent leaks.

Much of the department's water supply system will be beyond the control of the individual supervisor. However, in addition to immediately reporting leaks as they are noted, the supervisor can request energy-saving modifications that include:

- deactivating hot water systems of isolated facilities that are not used all of the time (conference room kitchens, for example);
- raising the temperature of refrigerated water fountains to permit refrigeration units to work for shorter periods;
- increasing the amount of insulation on hot water pipes, or replacing existing insulation with material of greater insulating capacity;
- installing spring-activated hot water taps;
- replacing existing hot water faucets with spray-type faucets including flow restrictors;
- adding water-saving flow restrictors to shower heads.

HIGH ENERGY-USING SPECIALTY AREAS

Two departments that are ordinarily highly dependent on the constant use of purchased energy are food service and laundry. The lists that follow are most applicable to supervisors working in those functions.

By far the largest number of items that can be listed for food service deal with the procedures by which employees perform their work, suggesting that how people do their work has a direct bearing on energy consumption. People who have worked in kitchens for many years will usually have developed ingrained work patterns that support many fixed habits. When energy was inexpensive and plentiful, work habits that wasted energy mattered little. Now, however, energy-wasting habits do matter and employees may need information and reinforcement to encourage them to change their ways.

Food Service

Training programs may be effective in helping present employees adopt energy-saving methods, and such programs are recommended for orienting new employees. Many of the points covered in the following checklist could be incorporated into a food service employee training program.

1) *General procedures and end-use instructions.*

- Carefully follow manufacturers' instructions for all equipment.
- Mark or color-code the switches in multiple switch banks to identify the lights each one controls. It should be possible, for instance,

to illuminate only a portion of the dining room when all of it is not needed.

- Schedule cleaning of kitchens and dining rooms during daylight hours whenever practical.
- Turn on equipment only when needed, and always turn off all possible equipment at night.
- Schedule energy-intensive cooking, such as baking and roasting, during nonpeak demand hours. Also for the sake of limiting demand, set a limit on the number of electrical appliances that may be used at the same time.
- Establish and follow strictly a schedule of preheating times for kitchen appliances. Equipment should be turned on at predetermined times prior to use and turned off at all times when not needed. Consult manufacturers' instructions for preheat times and temperatures.
- Plan menus that minimize energy consumption; shorter cooking times mean less energy used.
- Cook foods in the largest possible volumes; when practical, cook some items partially or completely in advance.
- Keep all cooking surfaces clean; accumulated grease and deposits reduce cooking efficiency.
- When keeping electric burners on during short periods of nonuse, turn them down. When actually needed, they will reheat in minutes.
- Do not turn on gas burners until needed.
- Fill cooking vessels according to manufacturers' recommendations; fill to capacity whenever possible.
- Use flat-bottom pots and pans with lids to maximize heat transfer.
- Cover pots and pans with lids to retain steam and reduce cooking time.
- Match pans with burners according to size; pans should be slightly larger in diameter than the burners on which they are used.
- Group pots and pans together on ranges; by using as little surface area as possible and adjusting heat accordingly, total heat loss can be decreased.
- Reduce heat as soon as food begins to boil, and maintain liquids at simmer. (Maintaining heat above the boiling temperature does not cook faster, yet it uses more energy.)
- Promptly remove the deposits from spills and boilovers to avoid carbon buildup that can reduce the equipment's efficiency.
- Begin cooking food in steamers when possible, then finish using the appropriate equipment.

- Use steam cookers for vegetables and starchy foods like rice and pasta; only small amounts of energy are required to maintain cooking temperature.
- Maintain temperature controls on steam tables to keep food warm without allowing large amounts of steam to escape.
- Do not load fryer baskets beyond recommended capacity; crowded food takes longer to cook and wastes energy.
- Drain fryers daily, and clean them regularly.
- Use low or medium flame for light griddling.
- Place food close together on griddle surfaces and heat only the portion of the surface actually used.
- Load heated broilers to capacity whenever possible to utilize entire surface area.
- Use infrared broilers properly; these can be turned off when not in use and reheated quickly as needed.
- Reduce charbroiler heat to medium after briquets are hot.
- Keep charbroiler briquets clean.
- Plan baking and roasting to use ovens to capacity; energy is wasted when all available cooking heat is not used.
- Use the lowest practicable oven temperature for roasting.
- Use oven warmup time to begin cooking, except for foods which tend to overcook or dry out.
- Load and unload ovens quickly to avoid heat loss, and avoid opening doors to look at food. For every second an oven is open, the interior temperature can drop as much as 10°F.
- Clean up oven spills frequently, and keep interior oven surfaces clean.
- Clean out grease troughs at least once daily.
- Clean rotary toasters regularly, and turn them off when not in use.
- Consolidate foods stored in refrigerator and freezer space wherever possible.
- Do not allow refrigeration units to run with little or no food in them; consolidate minor leftovers and turn off unneeded units.
- Minimize the frequency of opening and length of time used to open refrigerator and freezer doors; plan to put in or take out several items at a time; clearly label stored items; prepare schedules for the use of walk-in units.
- Be sure that items do not jam against refrigerator and freezer doors and prevent complete closing.

- Do not store anything near coils in a manner that might restrict air flow.
- Keep blower coils free of dust and accumulated ice.
- Allow hot food to cool partially before storing to reduce the work required of the refrigerator or freezer.
- Thaw frozen food in refrigerators; this process will permit refrigerators to operate on less energy.
- Always extinguish lights when leaving walk-in units.
- Schedule food deliveries whenever possible to avoid overloading or underutilizing refrigeration capacity.
- Close icemaker storage bins after each use.
- Use hot tap water for cooking whenever possible; a water heater uses less energy than a range to heat the same amount of water.
- Do not operate dishwashers with partial loads.
- Adjust power dryers so that the heated air delivered just removes the water from the dishes; drying by retained heat will continue after the equipment shuts down.
- Always shut off dishwashers immediately after use.

2) *Inspect and correct as necessary.*

- Through proper administrative channels, periodically request the utility company to ensure that adequate gas pressure is being furnished.
- Check regularly for shortcycling of automatic equipment and loss of temperature control.
- Keep all equipment door seals free from debris to prevent steam leakage and other forms of heat loss.
- Inspect thermostatic controls for proper operation; higher than necessary temperatures waste energy.
- Ensure that thermometers are properly calibrated.
- Check surface temperatures against dial settings by using a reliable commercial thermometer, and recalibrate or replace thermostats as necessary.
- Check cooking oil levels frequently; cooking with inadequate cooking oil wastes energy.
- Check cooking oil temperatures against dial settings to ensure proper operation of heating elements and controls.
- Thoroughly clean fryer heating elements at least weekly; do so daily under conditions of large-volume frying.

- Have gas burners professionally inspected semiannually.
- Check all gas units for uneven or yellow flames. As necessary, clean burners, pilots, and orifices with a stiff wire brush. If uneven or yellow condition persists, have qualified service personnel correct the gas-to-air mixture.
- Inspect for proper operation of burners. Ideal for a gas burner is a blue flame with a distinct inner cone. The tips of the flames should just touch the utensil bottom.
- Regularly clean burners, and ensure that all openings and air shutters are clear.
- Regularly inspect and clean the interiors of fixed well fryers.
- Inspect ovens for broken door hinges and cracks that allow heat to escape.
- Periodically check the levels of ovens relative to the surface they stand on.
- Have oven timers checked by qualified service personnel at least yearly.
- Inspect outside walls of refrigerators and freezers for cold spots; noticeable cold spots can mean inadequate or deteriorated insulation or improper operation of equipment.
- Maintain defroster units as recommended by manufacturer.
- Inspect the condition of all refrigerator and freezer door gaskets.
- Check compressor belts for condition and tension; adjust or replace as necessary.
- Drain and flush hot water tanks at least semiannually; accumulations of impurities act as insulation to prevent efficient heat transfer. In areas subject to heavy mineral deposits, consider the use of a water conditioner.
- Check dishwasher power-rinse for proper automatic shutoff when the tray has passed through the machine.
- Regularly check flow controls to ensure that the proper amount of water is being used in the dishwasher rinse cycle.
- Regularly check rinse water temperature.
- Inspect spray nozzles and tanks for hardwater lime deposits and remove as necessary.
- Inspect speed reducers on conveyor-type dishwashers; lubricate as needed.
- Maintain pressure-reducing valves in proper condition. Dishes will not rinse thoroughly if pressure is too low, but higher than necessary pressure will waste hot water.

- Inspect feed-drain valves weekly for leaking.
- Inspect pumps monthly for leaking.

3) *Modify or install.*

- Request review of lighting levels and, as necessary, prepare a standard lamping plan for all food service areas to use minimum required lamp sizes.
- Consider repositioning lamps to concentrate lighting only in those areas where people work or eat.
- Set duct registers to provide efficient air flow within the food service area and balanced air distribution between food service areas and kitchen.
- Reduce peak electrical demand by staggering the starting times of individual heating, cooling, and ventilating units.
- Place foil under range and griddle burners to improve operating efficiency of equipment and make cleaning easier.
- Equip walk-in refrigerators and freezers with pilot lights on light switches; these should be made to show outside if lights are on inside.
- Eliminate the need for power drying by using a wetting agent in the dishwasher operation.
- Insulate hot water lines in dishwasher recirculation loops.

4) *Other.*

- For all food service equipment, keep thorough and accurate records of all breakdowns, parts replacements, and regular maintenance.

Laundry

1) *General procedures and end-use instructions.*

- Operate washing machines and dryers with full loads whenever possible.
- Consolidate loads whenever possible; reduce equipment operating time by beginning operations only after all soiled linen has been assembled.
- Do not leave faucets running when not in use.
- Use cold water detergents when permitted and when satisfactory for intended purpose.

- Heat water only to the required temperature; hotter water than that required in patient rooms is generally unnecessary for normally soiled washables.
- Drain and flush hot water tanks semianually.
- Turn off the main steam valve when the laundry is closed.
- Run ironers as infrequently as possible, and heat them only when actually needed.
- Clean lint screens, exhaust blowers, housings, and tumbler baskets or cylinders regularly.
- Establish schedules to reduce peak demand charges; whenever possible, arrange to do laundry work during nonpeak demand periods.

2) *Inspect and correct as necessary.*

- Check all timers on washers and dryers, and adjust as necessary to prevent excess operation.
- Inspect water supply systems for leaks; repair as found.
- Test hot water controls; repair or adjust.
- Inspect insulation on hot water storage tanks, pipes, and steam lines; repair or replace as necessary.
- Inspect for steam leaks; repair.
- Inspect control valves for proper operation and general condition (including inspection for leaks).
- Inspect heat recovery equipment for proper operation.
- Check the front-to-rear level of tumbler baskets or cylinders; if the tumbler axis is not parallel with the floor, the result will be uneven loading of materials and significant energy waste (as well as excess wear on bearings and other rotating parts).
- Check tumbler rotating speed at full load; low speed will expose too little fabric surface to the drying air and thus waste energy.
- Inspect all bearings; lubricate regularly or as recommended by the equipment manufacturer.
- Check fan speed in tumblers and dryers.
- Inspect gas burners in dryers; clean regularly.
- Check and adjust the firing rate of direct-fired equipment. A higher or lower rate than that recommended by the manufacturer will waste energy.
- Check for proper and complete operation of water extractors; all water removed by extractors will not have to be evaporated by the dryers.

- Do not pull laundry makeup air from conditioned space; all laundry makeup air should be taken from outdoors. Removal of air from conditioned space results in a slight pressure differential that causes the infiltration of outside air into the conditioned space; since this air must then be cooled and dehumidified, there is a corresponding waste of energy. This should be considered whenever ducting equipment for makeup air.

- Investigate alternatives that will reduce or eliminate certain laundry operations, such as the use of bed linens that do not need ironing.

EMPLOYEE PARTICIPATION

Energy management will work best if it comes in the form of an organization-wide program with top management's enthusiastic blessing and participation. However, even in the absence of a formal energy management program basic energy conservation efforts can be undertaken and the supervisor can adopt a visible interest in energy conservation that carries over to many of the employees in the department.

Each employee in the organization is at the very least an observer of energy use and is thus a potential contributor of ideas for saving energy. All of what is desired of employees for a successful energy conservation effort can be distilled into the single, all-encompassing need for an energy-conscious attitude on the part of each employee. If the attitude is present, the rest will follow: active cooperation with conservation measures, ideas for saving energy, and observations and reports of wasteful conditions. The ideal situation would exist if each employee were to apply the attitude of a conscientious homeowner to the institution and behave as though asking, "If I were paying the energy bill out of my own pocket, what could I do to ensure that I was getting the most value for my money while satisfying all of my energy needs?"

Whether the employees of the department exhibit an energy-conscious attitude is largely up to the supervisor. As in so many other aspects of their relationship with the organization, the employees will largely take their cues from the supervisor. If the supervisor appears to care little about energy use, the employees are likely to care little about energy use. However, if the supervisor is conscientious about the amount of energy used by the department and pays attention to unnecessary use, leaks, and other losses, then the basis is available for encouraging employees to adopt a similar attitude.

As previously noted, the days of cheap energy are gone forever, even though the mid-1980s brought stabilization of supplies and some gradual moderation of prices. However, only a few short years ago many organizations, health care institutions among them, were faced with short-range prospects of fuel allocations and rationing.[4] The long-range outlook suggests that energy costs will resume their rise and threaten to consume a larger share of the organization's budget, that limitations in the supply of certain fuels will be approached, that controls may be placed on the amount of energy that each organization can consume, and that mandated targets for reduced energy consumption will be developed.

Even in the short run, however, energy conservation makes sense for the department supervisor. The organization's primary resource for the provision of patient care—money—exists in finite supply, and money expended through wasteful energy use does nothing to further the cause of patient care. Overall the individual supervisor may not be able to do a great deal to reduce the total organization's energy bills. However, a number of individual supervisors all thinking and acting along the same lines can change the bottom line for the better.

NOTES

1. J.W. Janco, R.D. Krouner, and C.R. McConnell, *The Hospital Energy Management Manual* (Rockville, Md.: Aspen Systems Corp., 1980), p. 1:1.
2. Ibid., p. 1:2.
3. Listings adapted from portions of Janco, Krouner, and McConnell, *The Hospital Energy Management Manual*, pp. 6:1–6:55.
4. Ibid., p. 12:3.

Index

About the Author

Charles R. McConnell is Vice President for Employee Affairs at The Genesee Hospital in Rochester, New York. For 11 years before joining The Genesee Hospital, he was Senior Consultant and Director of Personnel Development and Training for the Management and Planning Services (MAPS) division of the Hospital Association of New York State (HANYS).

He has written nearly 70 articles for trade, professional, management, and general-interest periodicals, and four previous Aspen books: The Hospital Energy Management Manual (1980) (with J. W. Janco and R.D. Krouner), The Effective Health Care Supervisor (1982), The Health Care Supervisor's Casebook (1982), and Managing the Health Care Professional (1984). He also serves as editor of the quarterly Aspen journal, "The Health Care Supervisor."

Mr. McConnell holds a B.S. in industrial engineering from the University of Buffalo, and an M.B.A. in Management from the State University of New York at Buffalo.